The
Body
Doesn't
Lie

The Body Doesn't Lie

A 3-Step Program to END CHRONIC PAIN
and BECOME POSITIVELY RADIANT ∞

Vicky Vlachonis

with Mariska van Aalst

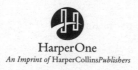

HarperOne
An Imprint of HarperCollins*Publishers*

HarperOne

HarperCollins books may be purchased for educational, business, or sales promotional use. For information please e-mail the Special Markets Department at SPsales@harpercollins.com.

HarperCollins website: http://www.harpercollins.com

HarperCollins®, 📖®, and HarperOne™ are trademarks of HarperCollins Publishers.

FIRST EDITION

Designed by Ralph Fowler

Library of Congress Cataloging-in-Publication Data
Vlachonis, Vicky.
    The body doesn't lie : a 3-step program to end chronic pain and become positively radiant / Vicky Vlachonis.
        pages   cm
    Includes bibliographical references.
    ISBN 978–0–06–224364–5
    1. Chronic pain—Treatment.   2. Chronic pain—Alternative treatment.   I. Title.
    RB127.V58 2014
    616'.0472—dc23   2013043348

14 15 16 17 18   RRD(H)   10 9 8 7 6 5 4 3 2 1

To my mum, Jenny,

for her love and light,

and for showing me the path.

And to my husband, Jerry,

for walking the path with me

Contents

Foreword by Gwyneth Paltrow   ix

Introduction   xiii

Part One: The Power of Positive Feedback

1   What Is Pain?   3

2   Living in the Positive   39

3   How the Positive Feedback Program Works   51

Part Two: The Positive Feedback Program

4   Week 1: Reflect   71

5   Week 2: Release   115

6   Week 3: Radiate   175

Part Three: The Positive Feedback Tools

7   The Positive Feedback Meal Plan   211

8   The Positive Feedback Recipes   223

9   The Positive Feedback Remedies   243

Appendix A: The Positive Feedback Questionnaire   259

Appendix B: The Positive Feedback Resources   265

Appendix C: The Positive Feedback Shopping List   281

Notes   285

Acknowledgments   293

Index   294

Foreword

by Gwyneth Paltrow

Deep into the third trimester of my first pregnancy, I drove out to my friend Stella's house in the English countryside for a weekend away. I opened the door to find that she had arranged a surprise baby shower, complete with my best friends from high school and college. Everyone had flown in to be there for me, and to celebrate Apple's impending birth. Overwhelmed with joy, exhaustion, and hormones, I burst into tears.

As part of the celebration, Stella treated us to manicures and pedicures, and arranged for an osteopath from London to come out and give us treatments. That's when I first met Vicky, a blonde Greek woman who looked like a modern-day version of Hera.

My friends were all jet-lagged, and I was third-trimester, dear-god-when-will-this-end tired, but we were giggly and teary, and so happy to be together. Maybe it was the emotions of the day, or the fact that the women in the surrounding rooms were so foundational in my life, but when Vicky led me away for my treatment, I felt safe enough to let it all go. After weeks of suffering from unrelenting back pain and anxiety about the birth, her hands lifted it all away, leaving me feeling light and at peace. I felt ready for the baby.

When Apple finally signaled that she was ready to come, I was so determined to give birth naturally that I labored for seventy-two hours before finally submitting to an emergency C-section. Battered and raw, I knew I needed some care—but my first thoughts were for Apple, who had been through the same epic struggle. In England, cranial osteopathy is increasingly administered to newborns immediately after birth, and so I called Vicky, and asked her to come and tend to my defenseless little newborn. Watching Vicky soothe and care for little Apple endeared her to me for life.

In the intervening decade, Vicky has treated my entire family, curing our aches, pains, and physical ailments (a strain here, a sprain there, a lost voice, a chronic cough)—all while instilling in us that physical and emotional pain are often one in the same. As I explain a malady, she'll always ask: "What is your pain trying to teach you?" Under Vicky's care, my pain has taught me a lot.

When I'm in a session with her, I'll tell her about the week's events. As I recount an upsetting phone call, or a memory of my dad that's making me sad, she'll press a point on my neck or my back or my foot, and I can feel both the ache and the sadness start to melt away. As an osteopath, she understands that a pain in the back is rarely just a pain in the back—it may also be a dysfunction in the ovary or the gut, the thyroid or the liver. And, perhaps more important, she understands that the pain almost always connects to the heart. She's taught me that fear can kick into your muscles and body, and that those are the moments when you need musculoskeletal support, the ice, and the strapping most—along with a cleansing cry on the table, followed by a good belly laugh.

More often than not, I spend my days bouncing from one meeting to the next after the morning school run, calling on all my mental resources to make the right decisions for my family, my businesses, and my career. This is always followed by time with Apple and Moses, where I need to be fully present, ensuring that they get the very best from me. By the end of the week, I'm utterly spent—and in need of VV love. In those moments, her voice, hands, and healing energy can pull me back from the edge of exhaustion.

Over the years, she has become an integral part of how my family functions: If I am out of town, she comes over to treat the kids and send them off to slumber with her magic hands; she stops by when everyone else is at the beach, just to pull me back into my body and help me quiet my mind. Like any over-tapped mother, my brain can rapidly cycle away from me—Vicky helps me remember that I have all the answers I need, and that everything is OK. More important, she's taught me to face the pain, feel it, and then let it go.

Because my house often functions as a midway station for those in life transitions, Vicky has treated almost everyone I care about. When friends come to hide from the world, to stay and heal from upset or heartbreak, I try to give them a quiet and soft place to land. I feed them good food, pull the blackout shades, and tuck them into a cozy bed. When they're ready to pull their head out from under the pillow, Vicky comes to help. We call her the Pain Gangster, Vickser the Fixer, Clicky Vicky—but whether she's carefully placing her acupuncture needles or working out a trigger point, she goes beyond the hurt to find the truth. Sure, there's always the superficial relief, but these sessions are really about the deeper work. Vicky will ask: Is this friend happy in her relationship? Does she need to slow down? Does she need to take her life in a different direction? Does she need to spend more time with her kids, giving them hot baths and tickling them to sleep? Over the years, Vicky has taught me that the answers to such questions are in the pain.

Ultimately, *the body doesn't lie.* When you hurt, you cannot hide: The truth will always push to the surface like a piece of shrapnel. At one point in my life, I had panic attacks, and an ovarian cyst, and issues with my thyroid, which all manifested through pain in other parts of my body. I'd been running fast, to put distance between myself and parts of my life I didn't want to face, and Vicky made me slow to a jog until I came to understand that some emotions can never be outrun. I had to stop, turn, and face them, so I could work through the issues, and find some peace.

My career has been full and rewarding, but ultimately, my family means everything to me. Vicky has helped me become a better mother: She's taught me how to connect with my kids through touch and positive visualization, empowering them to build up their little blossoming self-image in the same way her mom did for her in Greece. In her sessions, Vicky also harnesses the best from Eastern healers, connecting the acupuncture points and meridians Chinese medicine located over two thousand years ago with the latest discoveries about the science behind nutrition, endocrinology, and neuroscience. You'll find all of these worlds in this book, woven together into a simple, easy-to-follow plan for relinquishing the pain.

I love this book because I can hear Vicky's voice on every page—her kindness and her compassion, her strength and her wisdom. She speaks to me just like this, ladling out a mixture of love and brutal truth. The program in these pages details the same recommendations and homework Vicky administers in her sessions, and the same crucial steps: Reflect, Release, and Radiate. This book contains the exercises, meditations, and techniques we've done together, which together form everything you need to heal yourself. There are also some great little tricks, too, like a trigger-point massage for the bottom of your big toe, which releases the toxic anger from your liver. It doesn't matter what kind of trauma you've endured, or the amount of heartache, hurt, or toxic energy locked up in your muscles or organs—Vicky will show you how to face the pain and then let it go, so you can feel free and unencumbered again.

Introduction

Pain is good.

It might be surprising to hear an osteopath, a healer whose mission it is to relieve pain, say such a thing. But I believe that pain is a messenger and one of our most powerful teachers.

Pain is opportunity. Pain is potential.

Everyone has felt pain. Maybe you feel the lingering pain of old injury, or maybe your pain is the by-product of regular wear and tear on your body, a sign of getting older. Perhaps you feel a burning pain in your lower back, a tightness in your neck, a soreness in your shoulder. Pain can be the aching knees that keep you from running, or the carpal tunnel syndrome that makes typing up those annual reports an absolute nightmare. Pain can keep you popping Advil to stay two steps ahead of chronic headaches or crippling menstrual cramps.

Pain is a signal, a warning from the body that something is not quite right. You might think you got that kink in your neck from the car accident you were involved in last year, or the slow burn in your lower back from sitting all day in front of the computer. But if you look into that pain, truly *see* it, you will slowly uncover something even bigger: the truth about your life, your relationships, your work, your state of mind.

You see, *the body doesn't lie.*

Your body is talking to you. Those aches and pains you feel are often the outer signals of inner pains you're not addressing. All pain, every single kind, is both physical and emotional. And all pain, when you learn how to face it, understand it, and let it go, can help clear your path to a better life.

While Eastern medicine has tapped into the mind-body connection for thousands of years, recently Western experts have proven that the mind and body are not just "connected"—they are one and the same. Scientists at the University of Michigan did functional magnetic resonance imaging (fMRI) scans on the brains of forty people and found that, whether people were burned by hot water or looked at photos of people who'd broken up with them, their brains showed an identical pattern: Two parts of the brain—the secondary somatosensory cortex and the dorsal posterior insula—registered physical pain.[1] *The exact same brain patterns* occurred whether the test subjects felt a burn against their skin or felt emotional pain—the brain simply did not know the difference.

For decades, osteopaths and other medical professionals have noticed that people who suffer major traumas become more likely to develop chronic pain and inflammatory conditions such as fibromyalgia. Many of these pains are the result of a good process gone bad: When you experience an acute injury to your tissues, caused by an accident or a trauma, or by an invading pathogen, your body releases a flood of cytokines. These natural chemicals bring immune cells to the site of the pain and trigger your inflammatory response, drawing fluid from the blood vessels to cause swelling. White blood cells zoom to the area to help speed healing. Overall, a very efficient and smart system. Our bodies are truly miraculous that way.

Of course, this protective response against foreign invaders is meant to *protect* your body, not hurt it. But if those cytokines are triggered too often—whether through stress, a poor-quality diet, undiagnosed food sensitivities, not enough sleep, or, yes, even emotional trauma—the inflammation can become chronic. This chronic inflammation is thought to play a key role in, if not be the root source of, many dangerous conditions, including heart disease, diabetes, cancer, and even autoimmune conditions. If you don't slow down to take care of yourself, don't take the time to fully process and release trauma, the pain that started long ago from a broken leg or a minor infection may linger for years, age your body, damage your genes, prevent you from taking pleasure in things you once loved to do—and possibly even shorten your life.

As scary as that sounds, you have another alternative—and it's the only way to permanently release any kind of pain: You must turn and face your pain, seek to understand it, and then learn to let it go.

I'm not going to lie—you'll need courage to do this. None of us want to feel pain; we want to get rid of it. Right now, immediately. But when we don't take the moment to listen to pain's message and learn from it, we risk prolonging that pain and making it much worse. What you need is a plan that helps you feel safe while you dare to mine your pain—a program that can be your life raft when your emotional seas get stormy and can ferry you to the other, pain-free shore. That's what the Positive Feedback plan can be for you: an unsinkable vessel to a pain-free, healthier, and happier life.

Turn and Face Your Pain

I have seen a pattern in my practice: Many people recognize their *physical* pain and have no problem asking for help. They'll seek relief with a massage, an adjustment, some reflexology, a cranial sacral release, or a nice strong pill. But if they're experiencing *emotional* pain, not only do they refuse help, they resist even really *feeling* the pain—resist it with all their might.

Is this you? Maybe you're mourning the loss of a job or a close friend, but do it behind closed doors, never sharing the depth of your pain with others. Maybe you've endured and denied the agony of a bad relationship for years, even decades. Maybe you regret a missed opportunity, or you do anything to avoid feeling afraid or lonely: *Must check my iPhone for e-mail rather than be bored for one second and risk feeling the pain of sitting at this table alone.* Or maybe you simply try to block out *all* your anxieties and discomforts and fears on a daily basis: *Must have a glass of wine/hit of pot/tub of ice cream before bed, in order to block out the bad dreams and help me sleep.*

We can become addicted to these distractions—to anything that prevents us from truly feeling our emotions, especially those that are painful. And if we repeat these distractions often enough, they start to create very physically painful results themselves.

Perhaps your pain started as a physical injury—then quickly progressed to emotional when it began to disrupt your life. Maybe your pain started as overstrain—but why were you pushing so hard? What internal or external pressure was causing you to deny your limits?

Your pain may have started with an emotional or physical trauma, large or small. But what I want you to understand is that emotional pain and physical pain share the exact same brain waves and hormonal cascades, and these pain signals have the power to embed themselves in the tissues and synapses of your body and brain, long-term.

You may want to stuff down that anger and resentment of your boss, feed those feelings of loneliness and boredom, block out that fear of the future—but the whole world that you're carrying on your shoulders, that pain and fear that you're running from, that you're trying so hard to ignore, will find a way to bubble up, one way or another. And if you're not ready to acknowledge the pain of your anger or face your fear head-on, it finds a physical way out—via a shoulder injury or lower backache or a pain in the neck (literally!).

Consider the ways you might be hiding from your pain:

Do you eat your emotions?

Do you drown them in drink?

Do you spend all day working, working, working—never taking time to take care of yourself or your body, to rest and replenish?

Do you spend the night awake, staring at the ceiling—and then use caffeine to get through the next day?

Do you use your phone as a shield from the world—constantly checking e-mail, Facebook, Twitter? Does the phone feel like a crutch? An addiction? A lifeline?

Do you stay away from the gym or the yoga class, blaming your bad back or your injured shoulder—when you know that movement and exercise are exactly what you need?

Do you feel shame about your body and hide yourself inside, away from the sun and the fresh air?

Do you deny yourself the joy and pleasure of being alive—though you're not sure why?

If so, I understand. Trying to protect yourself from feeling pain makes perfect logical sense. After all, who really *wants* to feel chronic muscle or joint pain, let alone the soul-rending pain of regret or heartbreak? We use our little habits and addictions—overeating, overdrinking, overworking—like comforting Band-Aids on our adult boo-boos. These diversions may not make us heal faster, but they give us comfort, temporarily. The problem is, when we continue to rely upon unhealthy Band-Aids to triage ever-worsening emotional wounds, we tend to end up with *a lot* of Band-Aids.

Those unhealthy diversions—smoking, drinking, eating health-eroding food, avoiding social contact—start multiplying and just end up making you feel worse. You haven't dealt with the core source of pain; all you've done is add a dozen other sources of pain on top of it!

In order to live a life of health and vitality, you need to face your pain—all of it—and toss that Band-Aid mentality. You don't need a quick fix. You need and deserve *true healing*, from your nagging headache down to the bottom of your soul. And you can start right now.

How a Program Can Help

Structure helps us feel safe. Parents and teachers use structure to help kids feel calm and learn to take care of themselves—to brush their teeth, to tie their shoelaces, to comb their hair. As adults, we think we're supposed to have things all figured out. Even when life gets tremendously chaotic, we tell ourselves that we're *supposed* to know what to do next.

But life just isn't like that. In fact, life is full of moments when we don't have a clue what to do next, so we try to fake our way through. And the panic of not knowing the way—and having people see that we don't know the way—can drive us back to those Band-Aids. But I've found that having structure—a clear, step-by-step, daily routine to follow—can help you break the grip of those negative distractions. A clear structure can help you learn positive habits that ground you, nourish you, and help you grow. Structure simplifies your "What next?" choices and helps you feel safe from moment to moment in the midst of a very chaotic, very adult life.

When you have a map to follow, you don't have to worry that you'll get lost in the woods of your pain with no means of escape. Even if you resort to a temporary diversion for a moment—say you sneak a smoke or have a few too many glasses of wine at a cocktail party—you can always get back onto a healthy track simply by returning to your program. You don't need to be scared or to hide from your pain anymore.

With the Positive Feedback program, I'll teach you a step-by-step plan of simple daily routines, movement techniques, menu plans, and thought exercises that will guide you along the safest, most effective avenue for releasing pain. Think of me as reaching through the pages of this book to take your hand and walk you through the three-step process. Together we will systematically identify and reflect on pain-causing patterns in your life; help you let go of what no longer works for you; and blossom into an entirely new, energizing, pain-free way of living. The plan is designed to greatly reduce any pain-causing inflammation, increase your circulation and oxygen saturation, and release accumulated waste products in your organs and tissues. By the end of the Positive Feedback protocol, you will have developed an eating, movement, meditation, and self-care framework that will keep you feeling safe and strong and carry you through the rest of your life.

After two weeks on the program, you'll begin to shed unneeded weight, restore clarity to your skin, release toxins trapped in your brain and body tissues, and regain your vibrant energy and ageless beauty. By the end of the third week, you'll have learned a process that will help you boldly explore your core passions and identity as you design an entirely motivating, soul-stirring, and, most important, achievable path to your most deeply felt dreams. You'll graduate to living fully in the positive, okay with the fact that you are a work in progress, knowing that you may stumble into the woods of your pain again, but feeling secure that you have a map that can guide you back out again, anytime you're ready.

In the following pages, I'll share the program that I've used with my patients for years, everyone from working mothers to recent college grads, from members of the British royal family and Hollywood actors to international moguls and ten-year-old girls. Every single one of them, at various times in his or her life, was in some kind of pain. Some of that pain was physical, some emotional. Some acute, some chronic. Some these patients had been choosing to ignore, but ultimately decided to face head-on. Through my guidance and their own focused work, all learned to understand and then gently break themselves free from their pain. How did they accomplish this? They came to know themselves on a deeper level by tapping into an innate biochemical system we all share, a natural mechanism called Positive Feedback.

What Is Positive Feedback?

Your feelings impact every system in your body simultaneously. Let's look at why that is.

Your emotions are born in your nervous system—the system that physically runs up and down your spine and branches into every organ and limb and digit of your body. These emotions trigger neurochemical changes in your brain, hormonal releases in your endocrine system, bloodflow changes in your circulatory system, and airflow changes in your respiratory system. When working as it's supposed to, this integrated reaction is your body's so-called Adaptive Response: Your body meets a challenge (or stress) and, through adaptation, learns how to function better in order to meet that challenge.

As mentioned earlier, this Adaptive Response shares many of the same characteristics whether you encounter emotional pain or physical pain, and its primary objective is to teach your body to be more resilient, to handle stress better, and to continue to expand your capacity for life. Your Adaptive Response helps you become stronger for having endured a challenge. It's kind of like evolution on an individual level. Your own personal survival of the fittest, based on the "What doesn't kill me makes me stronger" or "Bones get stronger where they break" principle.

When the Adaptive Response is working well, it's a short process. You meet the challenge; your body's systems adapt to the stress, and you move on. Take exercise as a prime example: On a hectic day at work, you head outside for a quick walk during your lunch break. You push your body beyond its normal levels of exertion. You get out of breath; your muscles feel weak. But as you recover, those torn muscle fibers grow stronger and your lung capacity expands. Your body's Adaptive Response to the exertion increases your body's future capacity for strength and endurance.

You repeat the experience the next day, and the next. Because your body develops greater stamina, you don't have the same slumps in the afternoon, so you're not resorting to your diet soda at 3:00 P.M. Instead, you reach for an apple and few almonds or a cup of herbal tea. You build up to a daily habit of walking at lunchtime. The exercise helps balance your blood sugar and burns off your stress hormones. When your head hits the pillow, you fall instantly asleep. You wake up at dawn, refreshed and ready for a nice sunrise walk with your dog.

You've entered a Positive Feedback loop—each healthy, positive choice ensures your body's healthy Adaptive Response to stress. Each choice builds on another, making the *next* positive choice easier, more natural, and more pleasurable.

But Adaptive Response is not automatic; it relies on our good choices to safeguard the process. Let's say instead of taking that first walk on that hectic day, you choose to spend the same amount of time checking Facebook on your phone. Your muscle strength and VO$_2$ max, the capacity of the body to transport and use oxygen during exercise, is not only not strengthened—it's weakened. Your metabolism slows down markedly. Your afternoon fatigue pushes you toward caffeine and sugar, which raises blood glucose and increases the level of cytokines (those inflammatory messengers I mentioned earlier) in the body. That systemic inflammation makes your old knee injury flare up—your leg swells into a dull ache. Your plan to take a walk after work fizzles. You're still keyed up from the caffeine and can't fall asleep, so you toss back a couple glasses of wine (increasing C-reactive proteins in your bloodstream, another signal of inflammation), watch late-night TV, and doze fitfully until morning, never getting deep sleep's full cleanse of the neurotoxins in your brain or the release of anti-aging growth hormone that allows your tissues to repair. You are awake between 3 A.M. and 5 A.M., hot and anxious, tossing and turning. You groan at the alarm, or even sleep through it. When you finally wake up, adrenaline courses through your body—you're late! Your heart pounds on the drive into the office . . .

In this scenario, you're locked in a downward, negative spiral. Your body's response is no longer either adaptive or positive, and it can get stuck that way: in a dark loop in which negative emotions lead to bio-chemical changes that interfere with your body's natural healing mechanisms, which lead to less self-care, which creates physical pain, which leads to more dark emotions, which cause low self-esteem and in some cases lead to self-destruction—until finally there's a cut, tear, or break, quite literally, in the structure and function of your body. You have stumbled into Negative Feedback.

Instead of the Adaptive Response that builds your strength reserves and capacity for the future, your stressful, constant go-go-go choices trigger the Maladaptive Response. You might think you're putting on a good show, working hard, "staying strong" for your job or for your kids, but all the while, your Maladaptive Response is building up toxic reserves that will continue to weaken your system.

Finding Your Way Back to Your Body

So why do you slip into Negative Feedback? Why do you ever fall out of Positive Feedback in the first place?

In part, you can blame your wiring. Human beings are born with an innate setting that ensures we remember negative experiences. While evolution installed this nay-saying habit to help us prepare for the worst and spare us from repeating dangerous mistakes, it unfortunately also predisposes us to dwell in negative thinking and to jump to negative conclusions. When we're depressed, this tendency is further aggravated, and we can get trapped in painful thoughts and feelings. These negative thoughts then create fertile soil for Negative Feedback.

The trouble is, those long-lived mental habits trigger fear and leave a neurochemical residue—amyloid plaque, stress hormones, and inflammatory cytokines—that perpetuates the pain. And so the negativity continues.

Perhaps that's where you find yourself now: Without even realizing you're doing it, you're clinging to Negative Feedback patterns that cause pain and suffering because that approach is all you know.[2]

When you're clinging to your pain, when you're staying in the comfortable bosom of your old patterns, you're what I call "in the negative." This pessimistic outlook has tremendous physical ramifications and defines Negative Feedback.

When you're in the negative, almost every self-care choice you make—the foods you choose to eat, the way you spend your time, the friends you surround yourself with—is an unconscious attempt to hide from that pain. Your body has to deal with a lot, choking on all of these negative inputs for so long. Your body has been struggling to restore equilibrium, and the pain has kept rising. But it's hard to listen to the pain until you're ready.

But once you forge the courage to face it, you can begin to feel your pain (sometimes for the first time), work through it, and let it go. The very act of starting this process is your first step in entering Positive Feedback.

I have seen far too many people dragged down by Negative Feedback, separated from what gives them joy. I know all too well that if you stay in this state too long, it will ultimately affect your organs and cause disharmony within your body. Very often, a patient will come to me and say she's just been to see her doctor, who explained her condition to her in clinical terms; the doctor, I learn, talked about prognosis and medications and tests. But the doctor never talked to her about her emotions, her history, and where the pain began. If you don't take the core reason for the pain into account, you're going to be treating the symptoms forever—and you'll never get close to the root of the problem, let alone the solution.

You may need a bit of encouragement to face your deepest demons. But transformation begins with a realization that emotions in themselves are a normal part of life—they're neither good nor bad. Your anger or frustration can motivate you to make major positive life changes—a new job, new relationships, new courage to face old fears. Instead of allowing that emotional pain to rule your life, you can learn how to use it as a beacon to a better life.

When you're able to face your pain, acknowledge it, and release it, you're not only *not* weakened, you're tougher than before. You make the daily choices to feel stronger, sexier, more alive. You feel safer in your own skin, because *you* provide safety for yourself—you become reconnected to your body *and* your soul.

Positive Feedback is the clean, effortless, joyful state in which you take care of yourself because you want to, because it feels good. You feed your body with fresh, delicious foods and move your body in a fluid, graceful, energetic way. Your skin is clear and smooth. Your eyes sparkle; your hair shines. You are dazzled by life; you can't wait to cook a delicious meal, make love, go dancing or running—you feel like you're flying. The energy all around you is light and happy. You feel content and peaceful and optimistic for the future.

Perhaps you're so trapped in the negative right now that this kind of radiant health seems like an impossible dream. But know this: To rediscover Positive Feedback, you don't have to change your *whole* mind or your *whole* body right away. A few changes in how you eat, how you move, and how you unwind can make a world of difference. While it may take a bit of effort to shake off all the negative energy you've been carrying around with you, it doesn't have to take a lot of time. You just need to consult your Positive Feedback map and get back on the program: your clearly marked path out of the woods. From the very first

morning that you begin, just a few steps will have you well on your way
to the positive.

The Positive Feedback Program

At the beginning of my career, when I first opened my practice, I focused
exclusively on immediate physical pain relief. I saw patients with sprains
and torn ligaments, muscle spasms, chronic lower back pain, neck pain,
broken toes, fractured collar bones, severe menstrual cramps, labor pain,
blinding migraines . . . you name it. I used a variety of treatments—
massage, spinal adjustments, cranial sacral therapy, acupuncture—to
soothe their pain, and all claimed to feel much better. But the moment
those patients walked out of my office, I lost the ability to relieve their
pain. I soon learned that whatever my patients did *between* sessions had a
much greater impact on their health and the degree of pain they endured
than the hour they spent with me.

That's what inspired me to develop this program. Through many,
many years of careful observation and experimentation, I developed a
self-guided program that mirrors the process and the effects of the treatments patients receive in my office. The Positive Feedback program taps
the very same physiological and psychological mechanisms of each of
my modalities, triggering the same biochemical responses that I get
from acupuncture, massage, reflexology—every trick and technique I
use to short-circuit the Negative Feedback cycle. In these pages, I share
the same three-week program my patients have used successfully to end
their pain and suffering and discover a newfound energy and radiance.
I've seen, again and again, how this three-step process—Reflect, Release,
Radiate—can help people break out of their pain.

During *Week 1: Reflect,* you'll step back and look at the whole picture
of your life: What's already working? What still needs work? Where did
your current pain begin? The information you gather in week 1 helps
you face the reality of your current physical state, giving you critical data

that you can use to formulate your personal Positive Feedback plan going forward.

To prepare yourself for your transformation, you'll begin the week by firmly committing to the daily foundation the entire plan rests upon: at least seven hours of quality, restorative sleep and the Morning Glory ritual. Once you've started, you'll do these steps each day of the three weeks (and hopefully for the rest of your life).

You'll begin the Morning Glory ritual with a glass of warm water with lemon (more on this in chapter 4), tapping lemon's power to counter the inflammation in your body, regenerate the liver, and flush out any impurities in the gut. The smell of lemon alone wakes up my mind and lightens my spirit. You'll hear me reference this warm water with lemon very often because I think of it as my Positive Feedback talisman: No matter where I am, what kind of negativity I'm facing, everything gets better the moment I prepare and drink my warm water with lemon, my go-to mental RESET button.

Next you'll do gentle Tibetan Rites of Rejuvenation exercises, to encourage lymphatic drainage and bloodflow throughout the body. You'll follow a very simple but specific bathing ritual, and learn a simple gratitude meditation that helps you learn to trick the nay-saying voices and talk back to them. Then you'll finish your Morning Glory routine with a nourishing breakfast, to stoke your metabolism and give your muscles the lean protein they need for sustained energy during the day.

All very simple, pleasurable, restorative steps that I hope you'll enjoy and repeat for the rest of your days. (In fact, if you retain only one part of the Positive Feedback program, I believe that this daily ritual alone could make a radical difference in your life.)

Throughout week 1, your Reflect phase, you will also complete several exercises that will help you to think back on your personal journey and locate the source of your pain. You'll learn how to deliberately construct mental scripts that build you up instead of tear you down. You'll create a timeline of your body's life story, taking stock of the physical and mental pain you've endured. You'll take an inventory of your time usage and your eating habits, so you can clearly trace the time- and energy-depleters in your life as you currently lead it. You'll get the full picture of where you are now, how you got there, and what you're ready to release.

Once you've gathered all this critical information, you'll move on to *Week 2: Release.* This is the moment when you will finally let all that negativity go. With very conscious and deliberate steps—involving a specific diet, exercise, and lifestyle-detoxing program—you will tap into your body's Adaptive Response to clean out everything that's been holding you back and dragging you down. You'll flush the accumulated tension and pain out of your muscles and the toxins from your liver. You'll reboot your endocrine system, encouraging optimal hormonal balance to return. Allowing the blood to flow easily and effortlessly through your body, you'll let go of all the inflammatory chemicals, the lingering residue of all those years of hiding from your hurt, pain, and regret. In this Release phase, you'll clear out your system, turning back the clock on your body and your mind so that you can grow stronger in the spots you always thought were broken. Your catharsis will help you see very clearly that pain is and always has been your greatest teacher.

Once your Release phase is complete, you'll be ready for *Week 3: Radiate.* All the work you've done in the first two weeks will help you reveal a purer sense of gratitude for the gifts of your life. With specific meditations and visualizations, you'll stimulate your brain to reroute neural patterns away from those negative voices that no longer serve you and toward those that give you courage, strength, and boldness. Expanding from the detox of week 2, you'll learn a new way of eating that you'll continue for the rest of your life: a diet composed of delicious fish and roasted organic meats, seasonal organic vegetables, berries bursting off the vine, goat's-milk yogurt, savory nuts and seeds—all anti-inflammatory, brain-boosting foods designed by nature to help tamp down the debilitating processes that drive most chronic diseases, including heart disease, cancer, and diabetes. Now that you've made Tibetan Rites a daily habit and have added some gentle yoga and relaxing walks to your day—activities that taught you to move your body in a way that loosens up accumulated pain and tension—you'll start to plan for new physical and mental challenges that extend your transformation and the power of your Adaptive Response.

The Radiate stage is the time for planning for the future, reigniting passions you may have abandoned, deciding how you want to share this new glow of joy and gratitude with the world in everything you do—how you move, how you think, how you talk, how you eat, how you pray or give thanks (and yes, most definitely, how you look). By the end of week 3, your entire being will start to radiate, from the inside out, and you'll be looking toward the future with anticipation and eagerness to see where the path takes you next.

The Positive Feedback Promise

As you make these gentle, incremental changes, your body will start to climb out of the Negative Feedback spiral. You'll notice this movement in big and small ways. Maybe you'll sleep more soundly and wake up refreshed for the first time in months. Maybe you'll get compliments on how shiny your hair is, or how glowing your skin and eyes look. ("Did you lose weight? You look about ten years younger!")

Maybe you'll unearth your yoga mat and look up some new classes at the studio in town. Or start thinking about your long-abandoned business plan, or your dream of starting a community center. Your brain will feel sharp and quick—you'll laugh a good, deep belly laugh with a friend. These are all signs that you're starting to undergo biochemical changes that allow your mind to let go of old hurts and your body to more easily tap into its innate Adaptive Response.

As your inflammation decreases and you relieve your physical pain, you will feel more mobile and free. Your body will *want* to move: Suddenly you're going hiking and dancing. You're chasing your kids around the backyard and running behind their bicycles. Grocery shopping, socializing, getting through the piles at work—suddenly, everything seems easier. You've done it: You've fully entered into Positive Feedback! Your Adaptive Response is thriving once more, waiting for new challenges and new growth. Stick with your program, and these changes will continue to build upon themselves, allowing you to get stronger and stronger, keeping you pain-free for longer and longer periods of time.

I will be with you, walking you step by step through this entire process. As we go, I'll give you specific and practical suggestions for bathing, eating, drinking, exercising, meditation, and introspection—rituals and exercises that progressively build on each other and pull you toward ever-greater moments of strength and clarity. Take what you need, and leave what doesn't suit you now for another day—but know that, as I've seen with my patients, the more aspects of the program you choose to follow, the more dramatic your results will be.

Along the way, I will do the following:

- Explain how you can use your body's own trigger points to release negative energy, feel more relaxed, and improve your mood right away

- Share groundbreaking research about how quality sleep activates your brain's innate waste disposal system, whisking out toxic buildup that causes sluggish thinking and giving you a nightly anti-aging treatment.

- Provide recipes and shopping lists full of delicious healing foods that take little time to prepare but leave you satisfied and full of energy

- Teach you a five-minute dry-brushing regimen that will speed lymphatic drainage, make your skin glow, and help you to release toxins

- Guide you through visualizations and affirmations that help bring positive, protective energy into your life

- Share meditations that have been shown to reduce chronic pain levels by up to 57 percent

- Show you the physical evidence of the direct relationship your emotions have with your nervous system and your organs

- Explain how the Positive Feedback plan will have a long-lasting and powerful impact on the response of those systems and organs—a response that has been proven to help you live a longer, happier, and radiantly healthy life

If you've been struggling with pain for a long time, you've probably seen several doctors. You know that the symptom-by-symptom, specialist-by-specialist Western medicine approach, where everyone is focused on one overtaxed organ or one magic neurotransmitter, simply doesn't work. No doctor will ever be able to find the *one* right thing that will solve every single kind of pain: The *one* thing simply doesn't exist. Your body's history is complex—many systems have been working as one, reacting and readjusting to every experience, always learning and changing. But what you can start to do is see patterns—patterns in yourself, in your family, in your body.

No matter where you are right now, you can stop the pain cycle the moment you take the very first, smallest step. As you move through each stage, you will come to understand, beyond any doubt, that the mind and body are not just connected—they are *one*—and that pain is a clear message that cannot and should not be ignored or medicated away.

Wherever you are now, whatever pain you're feeling, the Positive Feedback plan will help you. You'll learn how to sketch out your own big picture so that you can start to heal yourself. You'll design a unique program to trigger your own Positive Feedback using everything you are—your anxieties, your cravings, your fears, your dreams, your passions. Perhaps most important, you will gain the strength to tackle the *truth*. Secure in your own skin, you will release the pain, once and for all, and finally move forward, with courage, with joy, and with radiance.

What is the story your body is telling you right now?

What is the story you would *like* to tell?

Then let's get started.

PART ONE

The Power of Positive Feedback

What Is Pain?

Man is composed of matter, movement, and spirit.

—A. T. Still, founder of osteopathy

Amy had just turned forty, with two children and a demanding desk job that created tons of stress for not much reward. In order to get herself through her projects, she relied on adrenaline-fueled deadlines and junk food. Amy never ate candy unless she was under the gun at work—which is just about the worst time to eat poorly!

Her neck was like a block of cement; her lower back and sacrum constantly ached. Amy came to me on an almost monthly basis, and I would do everything I could to help her—sometimes a spinal adjustment and deep-tissue manipulation, other times acupuncture and cranial sacral treatments. She would have a good cry and good laugh on the table, and then she would get up feeling better—she had had the emotional release. But I knew it wouldn't stick. She wasn't facing her pain; she was eating it, drinking it, working around it. I was giving her an itty-bitty Band-Aid on a gaping flesh wound. I knew she'd be back.

Every time I treated her, I urged Amy to stay in touch with her pain and to stop running for those inflammation-torching sugar treats. She'd nod. "Absolutely." Then she'd call a month later and come in for another treatment. Cement-block shoulders. Deep-tissue manipulation. Good cry (followed by a good laugh) on the table.

She'd feel better, swear to follow the program, then leave and fall right back into her bad habits. And on and on it went.

Until one day, a month after her most recent visit, I got a voice-mail from her. "Vicky, I *get* it," she said. "I finally understand what you mean. I need to listen to my pain. I've started to reflect. I'll let you know how it goes."

Her voice-mail ended there, but I could tell by her tone of voice that something had shifted. She was getting unstuck.

By the time Amy came into my office several weeks later, I noticed a change in her: Her skin was clear and rosy. Her eyes were brighter. Her face seemed to have more muscle tone. She walked straighter. She had even lost some extra pounds.

What had happened?

She'd finally heard her pain—she'd been *forced* to listen.

This forty-year-old executive, used to moving mountains at work, had finally been knocked over by pain. After a particularly intense work binge, her immune system had finally given out, and she'd contracted shingles. The chickenpox virus (the same virus that causes shingles), long dormant in her body, had been awakened by her overtaxed immune system and came storming out of her nervous system with a vengeance. Shingles sores consumed half her face, almost spreading into her eyes. The eye doctor had warned her that if it got worse, the virus might damage her eyesight.

The shooting and throbbing pain had confined her to bed for the better part of a week. Later she told me that as she lay there with an ice pack over her face, all she could hear was my voice: *What is your pain saying to you, Amy? Are you listening?*

When you're in Negative Feedback, it can feel like you're swimming through mud. Your body may feel weakened from injury or sickness— but, more important, without even realizing it, you're listening to a negative voice of fear, ego, and darkness.

You may be blaming others for your problems; you may be holding back, not sharing with others. Alternatively, maybe you're acting "aggressively happy," trying to prove your happiness to anyone who will pay attention to you.

When you're operating in the negative, you can't seem to make decisions. You feel like everything is on overload. You're scared to be alone, but also scared to reach out. You're living your life on autopilot.

Things can go along like this indefinitely . . . unless and until something happens: Rushing to the subway, you trip and fall down a few stairs. Or you feel a chest pain that scares you. Or you're suddenly laid off without the nest egg you'd sworn you were going to save.

While you're waiting for the ambulance or walking your box of belongings out to the parking lot, you wake up and look around you. You realize that you don't really know how you got there or what comes next. However, you also realize the most important thing: You are *alive,* and this is your moment of truth.

Whether this moment of pain and breakdown comes from a fall, a serious illness, a sudden job loss, or a bad breakup, I want you to see it as a blessing, a breakthrough. Sometimes we need a pretty heavy-duty signal to make us stop and think about our life. Do you rush around all day long, pleasing everyone but never leaving any time for yourself? Are you stuck in a negative routine, comforting yourself with junk food, not really connecting with your friends or family? Are you asking yourself those age-old questions, "Am I ever going to be happy? Is this all there is?"

Your pain—physical or mental, sudden or chronic—has arrived for a reason: to wake you up, and to remind you that you're a fighter, not a victim. To make you realize that you're alive, you're strong, and it's your turn to shine. The three steps of the Positive Feedback program can help you fully wake up, dust yourself off, and take back the reins of your life.

Our History Is Written on the Body

Emotions, *all* emotions, are normal. They're neither good nor bad; they simply *are.*

Problems don't start because of emotions themselves. The trouble comes in when you don't express emotions or release them. Layers of buried emotions build up in our scar tissue, causing adhesions in your fascia, the layer of tissue that stretches around all your muscles and organs. These festering, unprocessed emotions clog up your circulation and generally create disharmony within your body.[1] Once you really see and feel those buried emotions, and can pinpoint where the pain is actually coming from, you can consciously increase the flow of your body's natural painkillers and anti-inflammatory chemicals to help you release the pain and heal.

One of my clients has a scar between her big toe and second toe that she got over fifteen years ago, the night she broke up with an old boyfriend. He'd been the jealous sort: "Don't look at other people." "Do you like him? Do you think he's better looking than I am?" One evening, when his paranoia had hit a fever pitch, she dropped a piña colada on her foot and the glass smashed—and, with it, her relationship.

That point where the broken glass cut her—between her big toe and second toe—also happens to be an acupuncture point for the liver meridian, where Chinese medicine says your anger is stored. Research at the Mayo Clinic found that over 95 percent of these acupuncture points, which Chinese medicine has described for two thousand years, correspond to common myofascial trigger points.[2] So after using acupuncture on her scar to good effect in the clinic, I taught her how to use the self-healing trigger point of that scar as a portal to her own healing.

Now, whenever she is feeling overwhelmed or angry or she can't sleep, she will put her thumb on that trigger point and press until she can feel it "give," until the scar tissue softens and she can feel the bloodflow increase in her feet. At first, we used this scar to help her release the pain of her past. Now she uses it herself to unblock the pain of the present and to nudge herself back into Positive Feedback. (You will learn how to do this, too, in chapter 5, "Release.")

We experience all our feelings, thoughts, actions, and reactions through these connections between our nervous system and our musculoskeletal system. Consider all the parts of the brain that intersect when we experience strong emotions:

- The limbic system, the site of our instinctual emotional reactions

- The hypothalamus, which connects with the endocrine system and the gut organs

- The amygdala, where we process sensory information into memory and learning

- The cortex, where we regulate emotion

Every emotion we experience leaves a trace throughout these areas of the brain. Those exact emotions can be retriggered by anything we experience, whether in the real world (through our senses) or purely in our minds, that seems similar to those memories written into our cells.

Emotional pain is the same as physical pain—not just metaphorically, but literally. The body and brain process both types of pain in absolutely the same way. So while it may make perfect sense to you that your body still holds on to an old tennis injury or the whiplash you got in college, it should also seem reasonable that the pain of your breakup with your college boyfriend might still be locked in your tissues in the same way.

Those emotional and physical connections endure for years and years, drawing direct links between our past and our current experiences. Not surprisingly, researchers have found that people who endured trauma as children and still have lingering feelings of helplessness or despair have higher levels of inflammation in the body. Our early, unhealed wounds leave us more vulnerable to the many forms of pain, as well as to life-threatening diseases such as cancer and heart disease.[3]

We even carry the experiences of our *parents,* in the cells they contribute toward our growing bodies. Their cells migrate into every part of our tissue through our mother's placenta, nestling themselves in our lungs, liver, heart, kidneys, and skin, influencing our immune system. And it's a two-way street—mothers absorb cells from their babies back into their bodies. Imagine: There's evidence that the cells of a grandmother and an infant can *compete* with each other within the body of the mother, triggering an autoimmune response.[4]

We are all connected to one another, and to our past, and these connections are more than just words or memories; they are blood and bone. We haul our entire personal history around with us in our tissues and nervous system for life. Unless we become aware of our pain, we can remain befuddled and imprisoned by automatic responses to an event that we *think* we've long since consciously "gotten over."

Let's say an old boyfriend once, during a heated discussion, raised a hand to strike you—and you flinched. Or you once had a small car accident that made your neck tense up. Unless you found a way to release that tension, to relax that flinch, the original injury could still be impacting you. Flash forward a few years (or decades) and that same stagnant connective tissue that braced for impact remains stuck, frozen in time, dried out and cut off from healthy blood and oxygen supply.

Some of these emotional triggers may have been "installed" during high-intensity moments or as a result of unhealthy emotional patterns way back in childhood. Just touching these tender places can instantly recall the depth of the original emotion and unleash a strong stress response, a biochemical cascade that zooms us back to the core of that feeling, even if the precipitating incident was thirty years ago. Your nervous system doesn't discriminate; that fight-or-flight reaction feels just the same as when you were ten years old—even if you can't consciously recall the original incident. And each time old emotional issues are triggered, they leave brand-new residue in your organs, systems, and tissues—those systems that are all connected. Unless you can stop and face that pain, and work all the way through it, you will continue to carry and replay your entire personal history, over and over again.

Even today, now, in this moment, if you have a negative thought (whether conscious or not) in your brain, your nervous system carries the imprint of that negative thought directly to your spinal column, which connects directly to your heart, your liver, your ovaries—your entire body. We acknowledge that interconnection with our vocabulary: We

Which Organ Is Hiding Your Pain?

In traditional Chinese medicine, women's emotions are directly linked to different organs, as shown below. Where is *your* pain?

Table 1. **Organ-Emotion Linkages**

THE ORGAN	THE EMOTION
Lungs	Sadness, worry, grief
Kidney	Fear
Spleen	Anxious, over-thinking
Liver	Anger

talk about an insult that "hurt our heart"—literally, because the heart has more neurons (nerve cells) than the brain does. Or we refer to knowing "in our gut" that something is wrong—also a literal truth, because the gut is, in effect, a second brain. Our digestive system, from mouth to bum, boasts over one hundred million neurons—more than we have in our entire spinal cord, or even in the full peripheral nervous system, which reaches out from the spine to the tips of our fingers and toes.

These are established medical facts, yet many Western medical practitioners still seem to have trouble accepting that our bodies can register thoughts and react to emotions, in extremely severe ways, before our brains are even conscious of them.

I have a patient who is a professional singer. His entire career rests on a supple and well-rested throat. When that man begins to feel a tickle in his throat, he immediately fears losing his voice. "My God, I hope I'm not getting sick!" he might say.

Now, he might think that the fear he feels stems from the pain of an aggravated throat. But actually, the reverse is true: The pain he feels *stems from the fear.*

I have another patient who suffers from recurring panic attacks. She describes a feeling of "going out of my body" or "leaving my body" when the breathlessness and the pounding heart take over. Her mind starts to check out, wander off from her body, which goes into a gasping, suffocating spasm. Was it her heart and her lungs that reacted in panic first, or was it her mind that started the attack, drifting off, and the body simply reacted, trying violently to bring it back?

Some of my patients have endured pain for so long that their pain has become their refuge, their built-in excuse: "Sorry, my neck [or back] is 'out,' so I can't make it to your event."

All of these reactions are about fear—the fear of truly *feeling* our feelings, the fear of feeling pain. We do everything we can to mask our pain, so it accumulates, and then we end up using it as an excuse to avoid life altogether. How much easier would our lives be if we stopped resisting?

Our entire existence becomes more authentic the moment we learn to own *all* our emotions—the good, the bad, the ugly—in our sometimes messy lives. And that authenticity is the key that unlocks our body's immense self-healing powers.

Hitting Bottom

We've all seen inflammation on the surface of the body: You get stung by a bee, or you bang your finger with a hammer, and inflammation zooms to the rescue as local redness, heat, swelling, and pain. The cornerstone of the body's healing response, inflammation is the body's attempt to restore balance, to bring more nourishment and immune-cell activity to a site of injury or infection.

When inflammation is triggered too often by physical or emotional stressors, it becomes the default environment for the body—in other words, it turns chronic—and the entire ecosystem of the body changes. Your arteries start to stiffen; your blood sugar stays high. The cells in your brain start to wither and die. And when the mechanics of the body have been stressed to their limits after months or *years* in Negative Feedback, all it takes is one small activating event—twisting to grab something from the backseat, lifting a heavy box that's unbalanced, or sitting for hours on end working toward a stressful deadline—to trigger a new episode of potentially long-lasting pain. The sign that you've hit bottom in Negative Feedback can be pain, but it can also show up as fatigue, mood swings, panic, depression, insomnia, headaches, period problems, digestive upset, increased infections, and more.

When you go to traditional, allopathic doctors seeking relief, especially to "pain specialists," most simply ask you to isolate the pain and then give you pharmaceutical remedies to deal with that specific pain. I have no problem with this—but only as a temporary fix, a way to help sneak you into the early stages of Positive Feedback. Because while pain medication can be useful in alleviating the acute symptoms of pain— the blinding headaches, the joint and muscle aches—it does nothing to address the underlying cause of the pain. In fact, when you take the long view, pain medication more often *leads* to Negative Feedback than *delivers* you from it.

We've talked about how our Adaptive Response is the natural, innate way of getting our body as quickly as possible back to homeostasis. But rather than tap into this healing mechanism, many of our pharmaceutically based pain-management strategies seek to mask it—which interferes with our innate ability to grow stronger from pain.

In the United States, the most common reasons people visit their doctor are skin issues, joint disorders, and back pain; a bit further down the list are anxiety and depression, chronic neurological problems, and headaches.[5] All these are facets of pain. But the standard approach to "treating" these types of pain actually *keeps* us in pain—and in some cases kills us.

Research from the Centers for Disease Control and Prevention (CDC) suggests that our death rate from drug overdose has been rising in recent years, primarily because of prescription painkillers such as OxyContin and Vicodin. In fact, more people die of drug overdoses than die in car accidents—and 43 percent of all drug overdose deaths are from prescription painkillers,[6] more than heroin and cocaine combined.[7]

Women are most at risk. *The New York Times* reports that more women now die of overdoses from pain pills such as OxyContin than die of cervical cancer or homicide.[8] Alarmingly, deaths from prescription painkiller overdoses among women have increased more than 400 percent since 1999.[9]

Women are more likely than men to have chronic pain, to be prescribed prescription painkillers, to be given higher doses, and to use those drugs for longer time periods.[10] Likewise, women are more likely than men to die of overdoses on medicines for mental health conditions, such as antidepressants.[11] Mental health drugs can be especially dangerous when mixed with prescription painkillers and/or alcohol.[12]

Despite the billions of dollars thrown at the problem every year, medical care for pain in the United States seems to be getting worse, not better. The general population is getting older and many of our seniors can't take care of themselves. Boomers are less healthy than their parents were. Our young people are more obese and have a shorter life expectancy than their parents for the first time in modern history. And everyone is turning to pills as a cure-all.

These scary facts and statistics underscore the truth: Masking the pain only makes things worse. Instead, we need to honor the pain and try to understand the physical and emotional reasons behind it. My mission is to help you believe in yourself so that you can examine *why* you're taking those pills and ask yourself—once you've committed to the Positive Feedback program—if you really need them.

My guess is that once you've made a few small adjustments to your daily life, you truly won't need pharmaceuticals—or even want them anymore. Because the mightiest painkillers on earth aren't those found in a pharmacy or a hospital. No, the most powerful pain relievers are free, life-extending, all-natural, and in an unlimited supply at your disposal, twenty-four/seven. They're coursing through your veins every single second of your life. You just have to learn how to access them.

Once you learn to tap into your innate, self-healing pain-relief system, your entire orientation toward life will change. You'll see that you're not a victim of your pain—in fact, you don't have to be a victim of anything. You have the power to halt pain in its tracks, no matter if it comes from an injury, an illness, a heartbreak, or a negative state of mind.

The Master Center: The Nervous System

To understand how Negative and Positive Feedback control our experience of pain, it's helpful to have a better understanding of how the nervous system—where pain actually expresses itself—impacts every aspect of our health.

Caroline Stone, in her book *Science in the Art of Osteopathy: Osteopathic Principles and Practice,* compares the spinal column to a keyboard that "one could play—releasing various keys (joints) and improving function of the tissues/organs related to those keys—or as a mirror, each articulation acting as a reflection of the state of whatever organ/tissue sends signals to that segment." Osteopaths use the spine as a "decoder ring" to diagnose illness—they see and feel the body's reactions to these releases and we can tell how the organs are functioning even before any illness shows up in other symptoms or tests. Stone calls the spine a "window on the internal environment of the body."[13]

These reactions are related not only to the internal organs and their dysfunctions but also to how our tissues interact with those organs. If you have a knot in your tissues, or the bloodflow to a specific area has been blocked, all the healthy communication between different parts of your body will be disrupted. This communication breakdown can make normal movement and function difficult, if not impossible—which is when the system starts to shut down. That's the point at which people tend to sprain their ankle, or break their arm, or get those nagging pains in their lower back—exactly the pains that bring people to see me. Often those patients want the pain to simply go away, but it's not that simple.

The nervous system has many different parts, some of which are entirely beyond our control, and some of which we have direct or indirect control over. We have the central nervous system, which is made up of the brain and the spinal cord, and the peripheral nervous system, which houses the nerves and connects the central nervous system to the rest of the body. One part of the peripheral nervous system, the autonomic nervous system, plays a large role in the work of many organs and guides important functions such as our breathing, heartbeat, salivation, and sweating. The interplay between two subsystems of this autonomic nervous system—the sympathetic nervous system (SNS) and parasympathetic nervous system (PNS)—is what defines our individual response to stress. Rick Hanson, author of *Hardwiring Happiness,* calls the SNS the accelerator and the PNS the brake of your autonomic nervous system— together, they determine how keyed up and how mellowed out we are, both on a moment-by-moment basis and overall.[14] The SNS and PNS systems, depicted in figure 1, are highly influenced by both the amount of stress in our lives and how we react to it.

Let's look first at the sympathetic nervous system. The SNS is the engine of what evolutionary biologist Paul Gilbert calls the "drive system."[15] Evolved to get us ready for stressful encounters—whether eons ago with a bloodthirsty tiger or now with a worthy opponent on the tennis court— the Adaptive Response uses the SNS to raise our heartbeat, shoot up our blood pressure, and make us breathe faster. We experience a feeling of intense interest, and excitement courses through our entire body. This "drive" reaction happens when we experience challenge on the job, or take delight in our sport team's win, or anticipate a sexy date, or feel our stomach flip at the thought of the looming April 15 tax deadline. Whenever we need to hit the gas pedal and go, the SNS helps us do so.

Now, if triggered only occasionally, and for positive reasons, the "drive" response of the SNS can be fun and thrilling—our brain and body are motivated, focused, and rewarded with a natural high of accomplishment. Triggered too often, though, or in situations that feel dangerous or threatening, it becomes what Gilbert calls a "threat" response—one that is totally draining and depleting, and that hastens our downward slide

Figure 1. **Schema Explaining How Parasympathetic and Sympathetic Nervous Systems Regulate Functioning Organs**

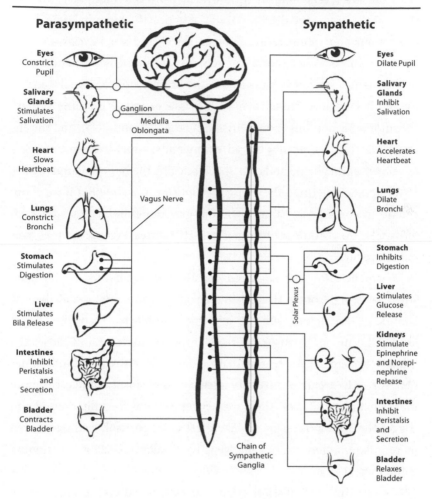

Parasympathetic

Eyes
Constrict
Pupil

**Salivary
Glands**
Stimulates
Salivation

Ganglion

Medulla
Oblongata

Heart
Slows
Heartbeat

Vagus Nerve

Lungs
Constrict
Bronchi

Stomach
Stimulates
Digestion

Liver
Stimulates
Bila Release

Intestines
Inhibit
Peristalsis
and
Secretion

Bladder
Contracts
Bladder

Chain of
Sympathetic
Ganglia

Solar Plexus

Sympathetic

Eyes
Dilate Pupil

**Salivary
Glands**
Inhibit
Salivation

Heart
Accelerates
Heartbeat

Lungs
Dilate
Bronchi

Stomach
Inhibits
Digestion

Liver
Stimulates
Glucose
Release

Kidneys
Stimulate
Epinephrine
and Norepi-
nephrine
Release

Intestines
Inhibit
Peristalsis
and
Secretion

Bladder
Relaxes
Bladder

into Negative Feedback. Instead of taking either the fight or the flight option, we freeze. Our nerves are shot; we become paralyzed instead of motivated. We simply don't have the capacity to sustain constant triggering of the go-go-go of the SNS, so the whole nervous system wears down.

The master control panel, the place where all of these threat signals come together, is called the HPA axis. This axis encompasses the hypothalamus, the pituitary gland, and the adrenal glands. All messages that travel through the body—whether from inside (our thoughts) or from outside (everything in the world beyond our thoughts)—impact the hypothalamus, the thermostat of the brain. The hypothalamus helps control our body temperature, hunger, thirst, and sleep cycles—as well as our emotions. When something requires our immediate attention, the hypothalamus sends out messages to the brain stem/spinal cord and to the pituitary gland. These then send messages to the immune system, the autonomic nervous system (including the SNS and PNS), and the endocrine system (especially the adrenal glands, which release the stress hormones epinephrine and cortisol). Basically, the hypothalamus issues an all-points bulletin to the entire system: *Hey, wake up!* But if we're not careful to consciously calm down and give our mind a rest after each onslaught, the chronic activation of our HPA threat system can take over our entire body.

When the HPA axis has been consistently bombarded by repeated stress, whether from a sleep debt, repeated arguments, a bad diet, or chronic dissatisfaction with our job, this high burden keeps the "hopelessness hormone," cortisol, coursing through our veins and causes the immune system to get swept up in a vicious cycle of stress and inflammation. A steady stream of cortisol increases blood sugar and releases more inflammatory cytokines. These messenger proteins then flip around and trigger the HPA axis *again,* releasing yet more cortisol, leading to even more inflammation . . . and the Negative Feedback cycle is functioning at full force.[16]

If we let this kind of stress go on too long, it can take a toll on every part of our body—especially thought and memory. We can start to lose brain cells, particularly in the hippocampus, the memory center of the brain. As delicate and complex as our brains are, their structure and function are exquisitely sensitive to the level of stress we endure throughout our lives. What was once a positive level of challenge can become a destructive level of stress if we don't learn how to handle these challenges in a positive and productive way.

And the brain isn't the only victim. When the HPA axis and SNS are triggered again and again, we exert major wear and tear on our cardiovascular, endocrine, gastrointestinal, immune, and nervous systems.[17] All that damage—and we do much of it to ourselves!

In modern-day times, especially in the West, we rely almost entirely on the SNS to power us through our days. Think of all the SNS triggers we experience in a typical day:

- The alarm buzzing in the morning

- That first cup of coffee before breakfast

- Road rage on the way to work

- The constant "ping" of your e-mail inbox, bringing more demands

- Crushing deadlines and demanding customers or bosses

- An ever-rising workload due to recent (or threatened) layoffs

- Road rage on the way home

- Murder and mayhem on the 6:00 P.M. news (followed by a dismal economic report)

- Kids screaming, laundry piling up, dog barking, spouse scowling

- Phone ringing with invite and added stress due to scheduling issues

- One last check of the e-mail before sleep—wow, so much to do tomorrow!

We not only rely on the SNS; we become addicted to its powers. Adrenaline is a drug, after all—we can become chemically dependent on our stress response to get things done.[18] And our addiction to excitement and stress and productivity—even when we're doing fun stuff—can become toxic and tip us into Negative Feedback.

Luckily for us, the parasympathetic system is there to help us set the brake on this stress response. After the challenge is met—project done; confrontation over—the PNS releases beta-endorphins that help us cool down, loosen up our blood vessels, and get our digestive system back on track. It's almost like pressing the RESET button. If the SNS is the accelerator that races us through a stressful fight-or-flight challenge, the PNS is the brake that slows us down to "rest and digest" and enjoy the fruits of our labor. (Gilbert calls this the "contentment" system.)

In a perfectly balanced system, the activity level in a person's sympathetic and parasympathetic systems would be just about equal. But in our stressed-out world, the dominant system is the sympathetic system. In fact, the response of our PNS, the so-called relaxation response, is swamped by the overpowering charge of the SNS if the latter is engaged too often. We must consciously slow down and breathe deeply in order to support our little-engine-that-could PNS.

Think about the overstressed executive. The multitasking mother. The recently divorced job seeker. The caretaker of aging parents. All of whom have barely enough time to tie their shoes, let alone wedge in self-care and relaxation.

While some people can maintain a naturally placid demeanor no matter what, and take time to decompress every day, most of my patients tend toward a perpetually keyed-up state of nervousness, sickness, and inflammation. I can feel differences in the reactiveness and the chaos of their nervous systems under my hands on the treatment table. Some people's energy nearly leaps out from their skin.

When you consider how many factors go into the functioning of the nervous system, it's no wonder that the potential for breakdown is so great. The strong and resilient functioning of the Adaptive Response depends on the various subsystems cooperating and communicating easily and smoothly. If you've been taking care of yourself and all of those subsystems speak well with one another, chances are your body will react to stress with the Adaptive Response—learning, adapting, growing stronger *because* of the stress. You'll remain in Positive Feedback and be able to bounce back quickly. But if your body is in a generally weakened state of Negative Feedback, any stress will likely trigger the Maladaptive Response,[19] causing you to move further into the negative, increasing inflammation and pain, weakening muscles, releasing extra stress hormones, and increasing insulin resistance. Whether your body treats an intense challenge as a breakdown or a breakthrough depends on where you are on the Negative/Positive Feedback continuum.

As we age, unless we're vigilant about doing everything we can to keep our body in Positive Feedback, our brain becomes less and less resilient in the face of these SNS/PNS swings. The very thoughts and experiences that rumble through our brain impact the structure and function of the brain itself; and with repeated stresses, we start to lose the capacity to regulate the Adaptive Response. The stress hormones coursing through our body interact with the weaker aspects of our genetic material and essentially age us. And that, my friend, is the ultimate legacy of a lifetime spent in Negative Feedback: premature aging.

Any of the conditions listed below can trigger, perpetuate, or be caused by Negative Feedback:

- An acute injury that was not well managed

- A deficiency in omega-3 fatty acids

- Emotional eating

- Environmental allergens

- Fear/amygdala overdrive

- Food intolerances/sensitivities

- Insulin resistance

- Lack of exercise/movement

- Leaky gut syndrome

- Obesity/toxic visceral fat

- Poor diet—one high in dairy, sugars, white-flour carbs, and processed foods (especially sodas, baked goods, pasta, fast foods)

- Smoking

- Unchecked addictions

- Unmanaged stress (both positive and negative)

- Unrelenting sadness

- Unresolved childhood trauma

- Vitamin D deficiency (caused by lack of time in the sun)

- Weak muscular or skeletal health

The amazing truth about the strength and nature of our individual stress response: Attitude really is everything. While most of their activities are involuntary, the SNS and the PNS are heavily, continuously influenced by thoughts. Every thought that goes through your head runs through this interconnected system and interacts with your body on a cellular level. You react to this information physically, sucking in oxygen, burning up glucose, crackling your synapses, and shifting your brain waves, surging your neurotransmitter levels up and down. Long-term, each of these changes leaves a trace. As you feel fear, excitement, desire, delight, and other emotions, blood surges into various regions of the brain, growing new brain cells, bulking up one area, atrophying another. Certain neural paths and connections are dug deeper; others are left to wither and die. Each of these biological shifts may even alter your genetic expression.

These ups and downs are not all bad, though. The enduring legacy of lifetimes of these surges and shifts made it possible for the human race to adapt to a changing environment, and they're the reason we've survived astounding challenges through the millennia. The reason we're still around is because our ancestors paid more attention to negative stimuli than to positive stimuli, a human trait. Psychologist Roy Baumeister called this our "negativity bias."[20] We're the great-great-great (times a thousand) grandchildren of the people who survived vicious attacks and raging storms, because they knew that danger meant they had to react quickly and keep those close to them safe from harm. We can thank our ancestors for being Nervous Nellys—they kept the human race alive, after all—but they also cemented the modern human brain's innate focus on negativity. Because of the strength of that instinct, unless we today learn to counter that dark focus, we soon discover that negativity can drown out positivity way more easily than the opposite. (Psychologist Paul Rozin quotes an old Russian saying that sums it up well: "A spoonful of tar can spoil a barrel of honey, but a spoonful of honey does nothing for a barrel of tar."[21])

Yes, we evolved and survived as a species primarily because we were constantly on the lookout for danger, our brain developing a habit of seeking out and fixating on the negative. And that tendency can get even more pronounced within an individual lifetime. If we experience a trauma, especially in early life, that event gives us irrefutable proof that our innate bias is correct, programs the developing brain to overreact to future stressors, and further strengthens our SNS's already heightened reactivity.[22] If we don't do something to change these unconscious instincts, our SNS continues to dominate and we become "wired to worry," gravitating toward fear-based, hectic, run-run-run lives. The chronic activation of our stress hormones ages our brains, our skin, and our hearts, and we get locked into the downward spiral of Negative Feedback.

Triggering stress can become such a default that our PNS can lose some of its power and become weakened. Luckily, we humans have learned that we can counterbalance this deficit. Hanson says we can consciously work to strengthen the PNS with, for example, deep-breathing techniques, meditation, yoga, and other centering, stress-relieving activities; such "work" helps us relax and allows the body to release tension routinely, before it can build up and become toxic.[23] For example, one Nepali study showed that a type of meditative exercise called pranayama can help strengthen the parasympathetic system in as little as five minutes a session. By slowly breathing in, through both nostrils, for four seconds, and then breathing out for six seconds, while thinking about an open blue sky, study participants significantly reduced their blood pressure and slightly reduced their heart rate.[24] This type of deep breathing exercise has been proven to strengthen the sensitivity of the baroreflex, a mechanism in our cardiovascular system that inhibits the SNS and activates the PNS. When we strengthen the baroreflex, we strengthen the PNS.[25] Neuroscientists, psychologists, meditation teachers, and even trainers for the U.S. military, who seek methods to help manage soldiers' chronic stress, have found that the stronger the PNS is, the more flexible and responsive this relaxation response will be in stressful situations—which is why strengthening the PNS is a major focus of the Positive Feedback program.[26]

While it can sometimes feel as though we're at the mercy of our brittle nerves, we *can* direct the growth and change of our brain and our entire nervous system. In fact, we do this in every positive choice we make, whether or not we do it *consciously*. When we opt to calm ourselves down, take deep breaths, meditate, take time to rest and replenish, we increase the strength of the PNS. We spend more time in a relaxed, contented state and our organs (especially our brain) get a break from their stress hormone bath. Our brain becomes less reactive to stimuli—we take a break, stay mindful, and thoughtfully choose an appropriate response to any situation. We start to fill up our tool chest with Positive Feedback emotional responses—empathy, love, patience—rather than reaching for the biggest hammer in the Negative Feedback tool chest: fear. By making those positive choices, we activate our Adaptive Response and nestle ourselves comfortably in Positive Feedback.

Yet we cannot become complacent. When, despite our positive tools, we make choices that trigger the SNS—focusing on the negative, surrounding ourselves with drama, not sleeping enough, or eating tons of sugar—we again weaken our parasympathetic response, encourage an increase in inflammation and stress hormones, and nudge ourselves back into Negative Feedback.

In the case of Amy, the patient I introduced at the beginning of this chapter, her pain was telling her this very clear message: *Slow down*. She needed to take the time to care for herself; to feed her body nourishing, anti-inflammatory foods; to get the full seven hours of sleep that her body craved; and to relax and replenish her nervous system instead of pressing forward, working harder, never stopping. She needed to reverse the cycle and get back into Positive Feedback.

During those many hours in bed recovering from shingles, she literally came face to face with her pain as a snake of burning nerves shot up, red hot, through her eyebrows, over her forehead, and under her hairline. Her doctor had told her that shingles among young and middle-aged people is almost always triggered by stress and a lack of self-care: "It's your system's way of throwing the fire alarm and really getting your attention," he'd said.

Amy got the message. All the encouragement and guidance I'd been giving her over the years finally came together. Brought to attention by a rampaging virus, she now understood what she needed to do.

She took out the packet describing the Positive Feedback program I'd given her years before. After reading it carefully, she spent an afternoon in bed doing several of the Reflect exercises described. While creating her Body Timeline—one of those Reflect exercises—she realized that after her youngest child was born, she'd abandoned the daily walk that had always kept her sane. She had always intended to resume her walks, but life had intervened, as it tends to do, and she was shocked to realize it had been five years since she'd exercised on a regular basis.

The next day, she started to do the Morning Glory routine and her Tibetan Rites soon after waking. After a few days, she felt stronger and decided to dive right into the Release phase. She threw out all her inflammatory foods and focused her diet on fresh, whole vegetables and fruits, green smoothies, and salads. She drank filtered water and rested, meditating under her ice packs. She started to talk back to the negative voices, to hold herself as gently as she'd held her babies, to surround herself in a circle of positive white light, just as I'd taught her in our meditation routine at the office. She threw herself body and soul into the Positive Feedback program.

And now, four weeks after being at the lowest point ever in her body's health, Amy looked positively radiant. I asked her what the trigger had been—what had made *this* time work, when at so many other moments in her life she had denied herself that healing. "The pain got so loud that I couldn't hear anything else," she said. "I finally stopped running away; I just stopped and listened. And now here I am."

In her Reflect stage, she realized that she'd been working so hard because she didn't feel able to say no: She put everyone else's needs before her own. Anyone who asked a favor of her got put to the top of her list—and she got pushed off the end.

As Amy dug down and reviewed the Body Timeline she'd prepared, she realized that the pattern went deeper. She saw that her intense focus on work had been draining her for years. That she hadn't felt inspired in many years—perhaps even decades. Her dedication to her corporation felt unbalanced, unfulfilling—even traumatic. And as she dug deeper, she came face to face with the truth: She'd lost herself, at seventeen, when her father had died and her mother had refused to send her to art school. A dutiful daughter, Amy chose a business major at a nearby university, attended an MBA program, and joined the corporate world right out of grad school. And she'd never been the same since.

All those years, those decades in between, Amy had been running from that pain. She *ate* her grief about her dad's death, putting on the extra weight to hide her sadness from the world. She worked hard at her job to prove to her mom that she didn't have to worry about her—but the hours toiling at a job she secretly resented took a huge toll.

When her kids were born, she poured all her repressed creative energy into them. She ran them to every artistic club and class possible, determined to give them the outlet she'd denied herself. She poured herself into them, fiercely protecting *their* creative expression—and all the while, the pain of her own forgotten dreams lived on in her tissues, coming out through her aching back, her extra pounds, her shingles sores.

But now, here she stood before me, a new woman, free and whole.

She twirled around, at least ten pounds off her frame, her hair shining, her body seeming to levitate. The very picture of Positive Feedback!

When I see her now, she tells me about her latest painting or collaborative art project. She and her husband downscaled their life to create space and time and financial wherewithal for her art. Despite a big shift in their income, she doesn't miss the old lifestyle; she feels as if she's finally *living* instead of simply *existing.*

Amy still occasionally has that tension in her neck—things get too hectic, the kids' rehearsals are time-consuming, her own art school projects are due. "But I'm listening, Vicky," she'll say. Her Negative Feedback breakdown left her with a handy pain signal: Whenever she gets stressed or doesn't sleep enough, or has too much sugar, or isn't doing enough to nurture her art, she'll feel a little tingle on her face where the shingles came out, just a little tickle at her hairline: *I'm here,* her pain says. *Don't forget about me.* But Amy knows that, even when she tips into Negative Feedback temporarily, the road back to Positive Feedback is just one step away.

Amy's shingles pain is a clear signal that she'll carry with her for life: a little warning bell that she's approaching Negative Feedback again. In week 1 of the Positive Feedback program, outlined in detail in part 2 of this book, we'll go through two exercises, the Body Map and the Body Timeline, that enable you to recognize the patterns that *your* pain follows—the physical outlines, the what and when and where of the pain.

Unresolved painful issues may be in your tissues, but they can be released. When I manipulate patients' muscles and connective tissues, I often help unlock the blocked bloodflow to those areas of the brain that are holding on to old, "forgotten" memories. Sometimes one adjustment and—poof!—that sad memory is released. But more often, you'll need to do more work to release the pain. I could massage those points all day long, but if you're not ready to face the pain and release it, no amount of physical manipulation is going to help. Reflecting on your own body's history will give you a place to start.

Once you know where your pain is, and the emotions that may have helped put it there, you can start to make other connections as well—such as the impact that your pain may be having on your organs or other body systems. Our bodies are full of trigger points that link to our heart, lungs, liver, thyroid, and other organs and glands—trigger points you'll learn about in our discussion of the Release phase and in chapter 9, so you can stop pain in its tracks and point your body in a different direction.

Remember: A pain in the neck is never *simply* a pain in the neck. Let's take a moment to help see how I key into my patient's pain and learn where it's coming from.

Locating Your Pain

Let's say you have a pain in your lower back. That pain may indeed be due to muscle injury or spinal trauma. Alternatively, it could be "referred pain"—that is, nerve impulses triggered by an inflammatory condition, a bone disorder, a problem with your adrenal glands or kidney function, or even a disruption in your ovaries or uterus. If you came to me for help, I would go through a whole range of questions to find out if the pain was indeed coming from elsewhere. I would ask, for example, if along with the neck pain you've been experiencing any other discomforts, such as diarrhea, fever, nausea, or recent unexplained weight loss. (You can get a sense of the range of questions I ask in appendix A, "The Positive Feedback Questionnaire.")

My questions and observations of a patient help me trace his or her pain through the neurological, endocrine, and immune systems—and to see how those linkages come back to the central nervous system. Osteopathic medicine teaches us, for example, that the sympathetic nervous system's connection to the kidneys is from the thoracic vertebra T10 to the lumbar vertebra L1. These codes refer to the areas of the spine that, as noted earlier, Caroline Stone said we osteopaths "play" like a keyboard. Don't worry—I don't expect you to already know or to remember these technical terms. Though they might seem like secret codes to you, these codes point to direct links with interior organs and tissues, almost like a treasure map that helps me get closer to the truth: *Where is the pain really coming from?* As figure 2 reminds us, the source may not be physical. Consider the common areas of pain and their potential physical and emotional causes.

Figure 2. **The Location of Pain and Its Possible Causes**

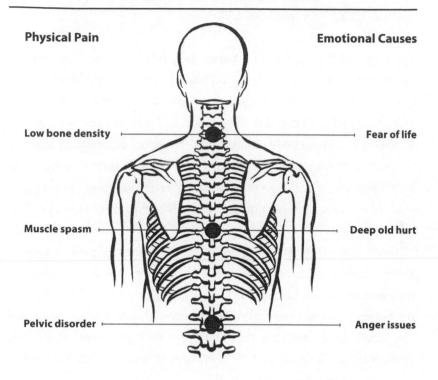

SITE OF PAIN	POSSIBLE PHYSICAL CAUSE	POSSIBLE EMOTIONAL SOURCE
Neck pain	Osteoporosis, disc disease, thyroiditis, parathyroid disorders	Fear of life, insecurity, difficulty coping, life overload
Lower back pain (in men)	Sciatica, prostate enlargement, kidney stones, colon conditions	Anger issues, stress of unsatisfying job/home life
Lower back pain (in women)	Ovary disease, pelvic disorder, kidney stones, adrenal fatigue, postpregnancy recovery, endometriosis, polycystic ovary syndrome	Loss of power, buried emotions
Acute mid back pain or pain at shoulder level	Poor circulation, liver condition, anemia, low blood pressure	Feelings of anxiety, palpitations, difficulty sleeping, fear of the future

Common Profiles of Pain

You may find that your pain presents itself every time you experience a particular emotion or reaction—for example, every time you feel anxious or receive bad news. That's because your dawning realization of that anxiety or bad news can link to an emotional memory that triggers certain receptors in the body. Because you experience emotion through the two-thirds of your body mass that's your musculoskeletal system, the trace memories of all those original and repeated emotions remain with you, in several regions of your brain as well as throughout your nervous system.

Every person's body is unique, and every person's pain is unique. Every person experiences pain in his or her own way. Yet as unique as pain can feel to the individual, I've also seen patterns emerge. Most of my patients—sometimes up to 90 percent—fall into one of two broad categories: lower back pain type and upper back pain type. Many have additional health concerns, but most come to me suffering from one of these two types of back pain as well.

Over the years of treating people, I've found that people with each of these profiles often share similar physical, emotional, and spiritual symptoms. Read through the descriptions and stories that follow to see if they resonate with you.

LOWER BACK PAIN

Lower back pain is often caused by muscle strain, too much sitting, or a disc problem. It can also indicate a problem with the ovaries or other reproductive parts, or the kidneys. Surprisingly often, lower back pain is food-related: When people have an intolerance to certain foods, eating those foods can cause inflammation in the gut, which shows up as lower back pain.

Think about how you've been treating your body lately. Have you had a diagnostic smear, swab, or scan recently? When was the last time you went to see your gynecologist or your general practitioner? Upon reflection, you may remember that you had an appointment just last year—oh, *but* you had to miss it to catch a flight and never had the time to reschedule.

Regardless of how the pain was triggered—whether by any of these causes or something else—you're now in an inflammatory state. Your muscles and tissue are crying out for help.

And maybe it's not just your back that hurts. A woman with the lower back pain profile might experience a host of really unpleasant symptoms—everything from smelly stool, to diarrhea or constipation, hemorrhoids, cystitis, and other unpleasant vaginal conditions. Often when I examine a woman with this pain profile, I realize that there's a connection to her fertility. Perhaps she had a difficult experience giving birth; a tissue-memory from this experience then connects her kidneys, ovaries, and uterus to the current site of her pain.

While any of the above-noted physical causes can play a role, I've come to understand that many people suffering from lower back pain tend to be repressing an emotional hurt from long ago. Their body remembers the trigger event both physically and emotionally, and thus their back pain may stem from that unhealed earlier trauma. If a person never deals with that deep-seated trauma, her lower back pain will return—and, eventually, may even get worse.

One of my patients, Sarah, had been struggling for years with fear and depression. During times of extreme stress, she would develop herpes sores on her lips. Recently, Sarah fell into a rough patch. She was so upset and emotional that she developed cystitis and bladder infections.

She told me she had lower back pain and tingling in one foot. After spending some time with her, I couldn't shake the feeling that her problems were related to the IUD birth control device she had inside her. At my recommendation, she went to a gynecologist. He tested her blood, did a scan and an ultrasound—and reported back that everything looked fine. We did a blood test and checked her C-reactive proteins to see if she had inflammation in the body. All those tests also came back normal. Then the issues start to worsen and spread to her bowels as well. She was in tremendous discomfort, and yet further tests *still* revealed nothing wrong.

We sat down together to reflect. "Sarah," I said, "we've got to figure this out. What is it? Why is your body bringing you back to that inflammatory condition over and over?"

"I'm not sure," she said quietly. "The doctor says this is all in my head, but it's *real*. Do you believe me?" I nodded, and I rubbed her back. After a few minutes of silence, she started crying.

Together, we retraced her Body Timeline. We talked about the fact that she had two kids, and she'd had a very traumatic experience after the second baby was born early, at twenty-nine weeks. She'd had to stay in the hospital for a time and nearly died.

When I touched her wrist, I could feel that her nerves were like soccer balls—they were banging everywhere. We did a Reflect visualization, and when we were done, she said, "Vicky, I think what's happening is that I want another baby. But I'm scared of what might happen, and I'm also scared we can't afford it." Her husband had just lost his job, but she couldn't get it out of her head: She was craving a baby. And she thought that her pain might be her body's rejection of the birth control device, the only thing that was standing in her way.

Over her gynecologist's protests, she made an appointment and had her IUD removed. The next week, she came in for a treatment. She said she still had a little pain in the vaginal area, but she felt safe—no panic.

Earlier, while we were creating her Body Timeline, she had confessed that she'd been sexually abused when she was young, and she talked about how that experience had devastated her sense of self-trust. When she was at the height of her pain, her doctor's words—"The IUD coil is fine"—reverberated through her, banging up against her own intuition. Once she decided to trust herself and had the coil removed, the pain, along with the stored-up trauma, was released. The morning after the procedure, she went to the bathroom and, after using the toilet, saw a large black pool of blood. Rather than alarm, she felt a tremendous sense of release and relief—as well as a restored faith in her own instincts. Another doctor later confirmed that all was well.

Sarah had a classic lower back pain type: a chronic pain in her lower body, especially her lower back, with some muscle strain—paired with long-standing depression. Many patients with lower back pain have deep-seated, long-standing fears, often from childhood. As they dig deeper and reflect, they can recall those issues from the past. If they're able to name them and face them, they can release them—and with those memories, the pain will often be released as well. Sarah's lower back pain had been taking her back to the past. She'd needed to face her pain to release it.

And following that release, Sarah's story quickly turned around: She and her husband agreed that they both wanted to have another baby, no matter what their financial situation looked like. Then, as if the universe had been waiting for her to release her fear, her husband's search for work suddenly bore fruit, and they were once again financially secure.

Sarah got pregnant within a few months of the all-clear from her gynecologist. Ten months later, after a full-term pregnancy and a blissfully uneventful delivery, she held a beautiful little baby girl in her arms. But perhaps the most wonderful gift of all was the internal strength Sarah built when she had the courage to reflect on her fear, face her pain, and release her anger. She had finally regained her trust in herself. She healed herself, reignited her Adaptive Response, and started living in the positive once more. Now she simply radiates with mother love—and her lower back pain has left her for good.

Your own experience with lower back pain may not be nearly as traumatic—you may simply need a new desk chair! But you owe it to yourself to find out for sure. In general, I've found that releasing deep-seated *emotional* pain releases lower back pain more powerfully than any other treatment.

UPPER BACK PAIN

Upper back pain, or the variant of neck and shoulder tension, is another common complaint made by my patients. The people experiencing this type of pain have to listen to their body and reflect for a moment:

Am I feeling anger or fear? Insecurity perhaps?

Could it be that the bonus I was expecting never came?

Does that make me feel inadequate?

Does it leave me feeling scared about myself and my family's future?

Does it leave me feeling out of control?

Neck pain and upper back symptoms tend to occur in people who suffer with present-day problems. Their emotions are typically centered on current worries and anxieties, which together have a compounding effect that ultimately triggers the physical symptoms. One emotion leads to another and then another, and the emotional pain and fear accelerate until they become overwhelming and finally manifest as physical distress. In addition to upper back pain, these people may have neck pain, sinus trouble, headaches, panic, flaky nails, and hair loss.

Do any of these symptoms resonate with you? If so, think about your situation. Sometimes these upper back issues stem from having endured something like a car accident and whiplash, and of course such things have to be investigated. More often, though, the pain arises from feeling unsettled, scared, or even panicked about life. Does that sound like you? Perhaps your mouth guard is your best friend—without it, you might clench your teeth so hard that you'd fracture them. Fear of financial loss may consume your thoughts; you may find that you can't have sex with your partner because you're thinking, "How are we going to pay the bills?" The stress of the present situation may be standing in your way of enjoying life.

My number-one piece of advice to people with upper back and neck pain is always radical stress relief and parasympathetic rehab. You need to improve your body's response to stress, and the only way to do that is deep relaxation and self-care—a lesson that my patient Adam finally learned for himself.

When I first met Adam, he'd just come from a breakfast meeting, and he was scheduled for an international conference call in ninety minutes. I had come to treat him in his office due to his busy schedule.

"Let's just focus on my shoulders," he said, his eyes on his iPhone as he did a final scan of his e-mail. "I'm really tight right now."

Tight would be an understatement: His shoulders were completely seized up, and as my hands worked over his upper back, I found several clumps of accumulated tension—what felt like years of blocked bloodflow in his tissues. "How long has it been since you've had a massage, Adam?" I asked as I gently removed his Bluetooth device from his ear and reached for my acupuncture needles.

"About two days," he said.

I was grateful that his eyes were closed so he didn't see my jaw drop open. Turns out that Adam had a steady rotation of massage therapists, physical trainers, executive coaches, nutritionists, chefs, and doctors coming through his office. A whole army of professionals constantly circling, on call to help him manage his stress level! At forty-seven, he'd recently been given a stern warning by his cardiologist that his blood pressure and cholesterol were dangerously high. His dentist had told him that he might have to get crowns because his back teeth were being damaged by all the tension in his jaw. Despite his legion of caretakers, Adam still hadn't enlisted the help of the one person who could make a real difference in his health: himself.

When I inserted the needles, I could see from the way they reacted that some of that upper back pain and neck pain was also masking referred pain from his heart. Working twenty-four/seven, always pursuing the next big deal, Adam told himself he thrived on the "rush" of business—but I'd seen enough adrenaline junkies to know when the rush had become an unhealthy addiction and was headed for a crash. That was Adam in a nutshell.

At the end of the session, Adam grabbed his phone and started scanning his messages. Without looking up, he said, "Vicky, I feel fantastic—I'd like you to come every day."

I smiled. "I'm really flattered, Adam," I said. "But I'm not coming back here until you do something for me." He looked up, dumbfounded. I guess he wasn't used to hearing the word *no*.

I explained to him that I didn't think I could do him any good until he slowed down a bit and gave his sympathetic nervous system a rest. "Otherwise, it's like using a water gun to put out a burning house—there's really no point."

I told him that I wanted him to do a couple of Reflect exercises for me, and I described the Time Audit and the Food Diary. I asked him to take a week to reflect on how he was treating himself; once he had that information gathered, I said, I'd come back and we could work together to tackle the Release phase and release some of his pain.

He took a deep breath and nodded. "Okay. I hear you."

A week later I came back, and we took a hike together—no phones, no Bluetooth—while he told me about his week. "It was an eye-opener," he said. "I didn't realize how much espresso I was downing—it's a wonder my heart hasn't exploded!" He told me that completing the Time Audit was the first clue he'd had that he wasn't sleeping seven hours a night: "If I'm lucky, I sleep five," he said. "But I'm usually awake in the middle of the night, my mind racing. I hate to waste time just lying there, so I get up and do something."

The hours in between weren't much calmer. The only time he had "relaxed," he discovered, was when he made love to his wife—just once in seven days. "Definitely need to work on that!" he joked.

We talked about his Release plan. Clearly, his biggest issue was his electronic leash—but what was he so afraid he would miss? And, more important, how much of his real life was he missing in the process?

Adam begrudgingly agreed to turn off his phone for three hours a day, in order to have evenings with his family and really engage with his kids and his wife. He also agreed to dump the white bread and pizza, cut way back on the espresso (he said he couldn't go cold turkey), and start each day with a Liver Flush Smoothie. He also agreed to make love with his wife at least two or three times a week. "Now that's what I call a prescription!" he said, grinning.

By the time I saw him the following week, Adam's shoulders looked about a foot lower than the week before. When I got him on the table, sure enough—his neck felt loose and some of the long-standing knots in his shoulders and back melted under my touch. He confessed that he hadn't told me about chest pains that had previously been coming and going. "I think I was in denial," he said, adding that he hadn't felt anything alarming in at least five days.

We ended our session with his promise to continue to look for more ways to disconnect and to baby his nervous system—and despite his still-strong urge to go-go-go, Adam has thus far stuck to that promise. Rebuilding his Adaptive Response is a work in progress. Adam is slowly but surely learning to value himself, even when he isn't dashing around making deals, producing, being "successful" every moment. He's learning to take a longer view and develop a new definition of success. He's also learning how to feed his soul with rest, relaxation, and health-supporting anti-inflammatory foods; how to connect with people he loves; and, most important, how to face his demons. Adam's upper back pain still comes and goes, but it no longer defines him—and neither does his work.

How the Positive Feedback Approach Can Make You Well

As you read through the descriptions of upper back pain and lower back pain types, did anything resonate with you? Did you see yourself in one or both of those stories? Are you starting to understand how the Reflect process can help you face and understand the root of your pain? Once you understand it, you can begin the work of ending the negative spiral and strengthening your Positive Feedback muscles.

For many of us, whether we realize it or not, Negative Feedback is an entirely voluntary state. We make conscious and unconscious choices on a day-to-day level that keep us in the negative. But our dissatisfaction bubbles beneath the surface.

Figure 3. **Positive Feedback Cycle**

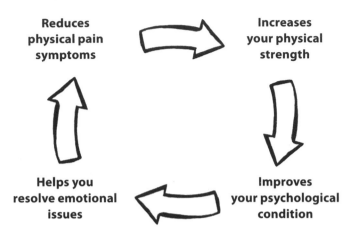

On an intuitive level, often even on a conscious level, we know we can't live like that for very long—but still we stay disconnected from our body and we deny our basic physical needs until we hit a breaking point. However, once we're ready to make a change, change comes thundering toward us with open arms.

Many people spend months or years stumbling around in Negative Feedback while their will to change is bubbling under the surface. All it takes is one moment to shift that energy. It's like the precise moment when hot water finally comes to a boil: We're suddenly ready to make the transition into the self-care of Positive Feedback.

The Positive Feedback approach recognizes that we are complex beings and require multifaceted approaches; it allows us to use multiple strategies at once, each one bringing us further into the Positive Feedback cycle (see figure 3).

If you're drowning in the negative, you can choose to acknowledge and listen to your pain and make it a transformative experience. As social worker and *Daring Greatly* author Brené Brown puts it, you can make your break*down* a break*through*. For every negative choice you make, you can make the opposite choice. As you begin to make those positive choices, your body will spend more and more time in Positive Feedback, waking up your Adaptive Response, tamping down your inflammation, and getting your body closer to its natural state of self-healing.

I was incredibly fortunate to learn the basic components of the Positive Feedback approach from my parents as a little girl. But even with my mother's and father's guidance, I didn't always follow the positive path—that is, until I had my own Negative Feedback breakdown. Let me tell you a bit about my story so you can understand why I've become such a passionate believer in the power of the Positive Feedback way of life. Maybe you'll recognize a bit of yourself in my story, too.

2

Living in the Positive

*Mindfulness should not be thought of as a technique
but rather a way of being. It is practiced for its own sake
and cultivated daily, regardless of circumstances.*

—Jon Kabat-Zinn

When I was a young girl, every night before bed my mom would sit on the floor with me, both of us with our legs crossed and our backs up against the wall. We would close our eyes and start breathing in a very deliberate way. In soft tones, Mom would say, "Think in your third eye point. And now, slowly, keep breathing in and out. And count: three-three-three, two-two-two, one-one-one."

My mom would then do a guided meditation with me, mentally taking me to a secret place I loved as a child, a beach near our home in Greece. She would help me to visualize myself carrying a younger version of me in my arms. In my mind, I would carry myself as a little girl and protect her, all the while saying aloud, as Mom coached me to say, "I'm strong, I'm happy. It's positive; there's no negative here. I'm the best." When I came out of that meditation, I had those positive thoughts in my head as I drifted off to sleep.

Mom and I did this practice for years and years. I could *feel* that it helped me, and that intuition is now supported by science. Researchers now know that meditation lowers blood pressure, decreases risk of depression and anxiety, improves immune-system function, and lowers pain sensitivity. Brown University scientists believe that meditation works because it allows a person to gain control over certain alpha brain rhythms that manage how the brain processes and filters sensations and thoughts, including pain and sad memories.[1] Even just brief bouts of meditation can change the very structure of your brain in ways that can eventually help you become more engaged with the current moment, more content and grateful for your blessings, and more empathetic to the struggles and triumphs of other people.

Of course, Mom didn't know about the cutting-edge neuroscience that would prove the benefits of meditation decades later; she was simply following her intuition. She knew on some level that our thoughts create our reality. To this day I'm still reaping the benefits of those early meditations and the strength I got from my mom.

When you start from a place of safety and confidence, you are equipped with skills that help you tackle any challenge. Whether or not your parents loved you, whether you grew up within a dysfunctional family dynamic, whether you ate fresh whole foods or lots of processed foods, whether or not you were encouraged to enjoy moving your body—all these issues factor into the resilience of your Adaptive Response, the ability of your body to rebound from stress in a positive way. A stable foundation allows you to maintain a healthy state more easily and for longer periods of time. But an unstable foundation left over from your formative years can perpetuate emotional pain and create physical pain—the kind of pain that brings many patients to my office—until you can learn a *new* way..

In many ways, I feel as if I were born to do this work. While I was growing up, Dad traveled to Australia and America, teaching tennis professionally for the Greek national team and setting up tennis camps. Sometimes we'd travel as a whole family and stay at the camp together all summer. Dad would teach tennis, mom would teach yoga, and we'd have a free holiday. Along with yoga, Mom taught classes on nutrition and was a massage therapist. She was a budding health guru at a time when those kinds of ideas were just starting to catch on in Greece. She had full faith in the mind's ability to heal and control the body.

My positive relationship with my parents helped me to avoid many of the challenging problems young women encounter with fear or a lack of self-confidence. Surprisingly, though, it was this strong connection with my family that was a root cause of my first health crisis.

My grandmother was always there for us. I used to go to her house on the weekends, and I loved being there. Every time we visited, she spent hours in the kitchen. My mom would say, "Grandma is baking this cake with love for us." And while I understood the spirit of what she was saying, those cakes from Grandma didn't love my body in return. In fact, those cakes taught me a huge lesson about the power of foods to hurt—and to heal.

Grandma made her living by cooking. When I went to her house or visited her at one of the hotels on the Greek islands where she worked, I had multiple helpings of the big carrot cakes, orange cakes, and other goodies that she baked up. And then I would go home and get sick. The first time this happened I was sixteen, but it took a while before I finally made the connection: Every time I went to Granny's house and ate those Greek cheese pies with all that cow's milk and drank all that orange juice, I would end up with cold sores and eczema.

My mom had always made sure we ate extremely health-promoting food at home. A sugar treat was a major deal. ("It's your birthday—oh, okay, you're allowed a birthday cake.") We would eat "naughty" things only at Grandma's. Although Grandma had her own fruit and vegetables growing in the back garden, and she produced her own honey and olive oil, she always felt that we needed a treat. She was up early, at 4:00 or 5:00 A.M., cooking cakes and pies for our *breakfast*.

My mom knew that this gave her own mother tremendous pleasure. Food was love for Granny, and Mom wouldn't dream of forbidding her mom to bake for me. What Mom did instead was help me understand what the food was doing to *me*.

One method Mom used might surprise you: She weighed me every day. She didn't do this to shame me. On the contrary, my weight range was essential health information, data that could help me get more in tune with changes in my body. As we stood together in the bathroom, Mom taught me a whole regimen. I was to look at myself in the mirror every day, then weigh myself, then use a dry brush all over my body—all practices I've been doing every day for over twenty years.

I didn't know then how much of an impact this ritual would have on my life. Back then I was just doing as I was told. Now, though, I credit my mom with helping me know and listen to my body. The daily regimen has given me a close and vital connection to the daily ebbs and flows of my body. Doing the ritual every morning is like getting a status report on my body's journey on the continuum between Positive and Negative Feedback.

Early on, I didn't make (or didn't want to make) the connection that the foods I was eating at my grandmother's house were making me feel bad. Whenever Grandma found out that I was feeling sick, she insisted that I drink orange juice to make me feel better.

Bigger cold sores. More yummy cake.

My mom would simply state the facts. "Vicky, you've come back from Grandma's and you've got cold sores." I would wake up with neck pain and Mom would say, "You're bloated and you've gained two kilos. What did you eat?" Well, pizza, pasta, spinach pie, and cheese pie, Mom—why do you ask?

Seems like a joke to me now—how could I not have seen the connection? All that dairy and refined flour (pizza, pasta, pies) was acidifying my system and triggering an inflammatory response that came out in cold sores, eczema, and bloating. It wasn't until I got older that I realized that food made a huge day-to-day difference in how I felt. *The body doesn't lie.*

Fortunately, my mom knew what I was going through—not just the obvious things like my gaining weight or getting cold sores, but how I *felt*. The thing that had inspired her to learn about nutrition years earlier had been the intestinal problems she'd endured while growing up with the same diet that was now plaguing me.

Like her, I wanted to be a healer. And like her, I had to learn to treat myself first. But I didn't fully realize how important nutrition was until I was twenty-two or twenty-three—and those yummy cakes were starting to seriously threaten my long-term health.

In 1993 I traveled to London to study to be an osteopath, first at the British School of Osteopathy, then at the European School of Osteopathy, where I was one of the first women to receive a master of science degree. A form of "manual therapy" that centers on the relationship between the structure and function of the body, osteopathy doesn't use surgery or drugs, but instead taps into the body's own self-healing mechanisms to treat illness and disease. I was drawn to holistic osteopathy because it's about the *whole* body. I studied the research behind everything I'd learned at home: To be strong, you must exercise; for strong, pain-free muscles, you have to avoid certain foods; to be healthy and happy, you have to look after your mental and spiritual health.

I had been brought up with all those elements, and was thrilled to find a career that would combine my passions and my work. I couldn't get enough: While I was busy with my studies, I was also meeting nutritionists, homeopaths, and Chinese herbalists, and immersing myself in the fascinating world of integrated medicine.

Yet—and you might think this is crazy—even while I was studying osteopathy, learning all these things, I was *still* going to my grandmother's whenever I was back in Greece, and eating lots of cakes and sweets. Clearly, I still hadn't *truly* made the connection. I certainly recognized good nutrition as the ideal, but it wasn't until I endured major pain that I really changed my diet, and my life, forever.

The Turnaround

My problems started with lower back pain and knee pain. I was gutting it out through long days and nights, taking classes, learning how to treat patients. I lived on diet soda and sugar-filled yogurt. At the end of each long day, my lower back would ache and my knees felt like they belonged to a sixty-year-old woman, not a vital woman in her early twenties.

Gradually, I also began to feel a dull ache in my lower abdomen that became more regular and more intense.

I lived with the aches and pains, and their increasing intensity, for about a year before I went to get them checked out. My general practitioner from the National Health Service in London gave me a cursory going-over, told me that I was constipated and bloated, and sent me home with a prescription for stool softener.

I knew the problem was much bigger; this wasn't going to help me. Finally, I did what I should have done months earlier: I called my mom.

"Vicky, please just fly to Greece tomorrow," she pleaded. She wanted to take me to her father's friend, an ob-gyn my mom had known her whole life. Grateful for her help, I hung up and bought my plane ticket.

Sitting in his office two days later, I learned where the pain was coming from. "Wow, you're either four months pregnant, or you have a huge cyst," he said, after examining me. "Let's jump in my car right away. If you were my daughter, I would trust only one colleague—he's an expert in laparoscopy. I'll get you in to see him." He shook his head. "If he can't do it, I'll need to operate on you myself. I don't want you to lose an ovary."

The treatment moved very quickly. The laparoscopic expert operated on me the next morning, and the cyst was removed. That wasn't the end, though. During surgery, he discovered that I had other, smaller cysts. The two doctors agreed that they needed me to undergo a special medical treatment to stop my periods for five or six months. "You must have some injections; they're very important," the doctor and family friend said. "These hormones will mess you up emotionally, but there's no other way. We don't want those other cysts to grow."

What followed was one of the most difficult times in my life, thanks to those injections. I had night sweats along with emotional ups and downs. I had menopausal symptoms at twenty-three years old! When I returned to the doctor, thanks to the hormone shots, the endometrial cysts were gone. But the doctor was certain: I had polycystic ovary syndrome, or PCOS.

"Vicky, I'm sorry, but we can't get rid of these—they'll just keep coming back," the doctor said. "You have to go on the Pill."

I was scared. I didn't want to go back to those night sweats and that emotional roller coaster. My mother knew I didn't want to take the Pill—the hormones had really messed with my life when the doctor had tried them earlier, and I wasn't eager to be on them every day—so she thought about other options.

"Well, hold on, Vicky," she said. "What about that person who did a study on endometriosis? Check out what he said about a food sensitivity diet. You love your dairy and sugar, but maybe they're triggering the cysts. What about stopping them? Maybe we should request a food sensitivity blood test."

Mom was, again, far ahead of her time. Everyone knew about allergies, but not many people had heard about food sensitivities in the eighties and nineties. Mom, though, had been avoiding common trigger foods for my entire life. I'd been brought up in a nearly pristine food environment, thanks to her—but those lessons had left me as soon as I left home. I'd gone to university and fallen into most of the same bad habits as my fellow students. I was depending on diet soda and Kit-Kats to power me through late nights of studying. As a result, the same things were happening to me at school that had often happened to me in Grandma's kitchen.

We had the testing done, and when I saw the results, I finally had proof that the dairy, wheat, sugar, and other foods were giving me eczema, allergies, skin problems—and now PCOS. I tried my mother's advice: to dry out my system and stick to a nonreactive diet. I knew I needed to do *something,* and her approach seemed as good as any.

Six months later, I went back to our family friend, the Greek ob-gyn. He was elated. "Hey, all the cysts are gone! You must've been taking the birth control pills after all!"

I said, "Well, no—I've done this diet, and . . ."

I started telling him about food sensitivity and inflammation, and avoiding wheat, sugar, oranges, and balsamic vinegar. I wanted to share with him that I'd gone to see an acupuncturist, a nutritionist, a reflexologist, and a cranial osteopath.

He held his hand up almost immediately. He couldn't wait to cut me off. "Well, you go ahead and do your witch doctor stuff or whatever you call it. Your magic food stuff." He shook his head and muttered to himself.

I respected him—he had saved my ovary!—so his dismissal stung. But only for a second—and after that, his reaction strengthened my resolve to study these other fields. I'd been studying the research, and now I'd seen and felt firsthand what these other modalities could do. Now it was my turn to help let the world know how much of a difference alternative approaches could make, not only helping people feel healthy on a regular basis, but also providing drastic improvement in the face of a painful health condition.

I sometimes still see this kind of knee-jerk negativity when I mention the power of food to my patients. That's always the best time to tell them my story: that I healed my PCOS with food. PCOS afflicts between 5 and 10 percent of young women, sometimes as young as eleven years old. Until we find the cause and the cure for PCOS, the only medical treatment being used to manage symptoms is the birth control pill. Many women would gladly avoid the Pill if they could, so I tell them that a nutritional approach worked for me, and most have to admit that healing themselves with food seems like a pretty good deal.

Pain is a tremendous teacher. Pain is an urgent message that we're not living the lives we should be. Pain is a signal that points to our past—and urges us toward the future. My own pain became my internal compass, pointing me in the direction I needed to go. I developed the Positive Feedback program so that you could have the same kind of epiphany, so that you could learn how to understand your own pain, read its signals, and use it as a map toward a better life.

The pain that I felt with that large cyst was really the turning point in my life as a healer. Before that, my eczema and constipation had been uncomfortable—but they weren't enough to *change* me. I had the cold sores, sure—but the connection hadn't really sunk in yet. I was still young. Mom had told me when I was sixteen, but I didn't listen. But the first large cyst—that was a big deal. That lower back pain was my signal, my message—and I finally realized it was time to pay attention.

The worst cyst was seven centimeters in diameter. After the surgery, the doctor said, "We've just removed a big orange." (Which was a cheeky joke from my body, because I clearly had developed a sensitivity to oranges!)

My new patients sometimes ask me, "Why do you do this diet? Why are you so strict? Don't you ever want to go and eat a big hamburger and a big chocolate cake with whipped cream?"

The simple truth is that now I truly *don't* want to eat those foods. Healthy eating has become a part of life for me. At one point, the thought of never having Grandma's orange cake again might have made me cry. But now, eating in a way that keeps me in Positive Feedback has become easy and joyful. I still like cake on special occasions—but now I choose gluten-free and Stevia-sweetened versions instead, because I know they treat my body better.

I love teaching people about eating things that are just as tasty as those that are bad for us, and that have the added bonus of anti-inflammatory properties. Foods that heal make all the difference. Your diet is your foundation. When you eat bad foods, you're not feeding your body; you're feeding bad bacteria, intestinal worms, and systemic inflammation.

You're also feeding into Negative Feedback. When I finally learned this lesson, it changed every single thing in my life.

Analyzing the Whole Picture

When my training was complete and I started seeing patients, I worked in the Royal Ballet School, treating the cast members of *The Lion King*, *Cats*, and other shows in London's West End. My focus was strictly musculoskeletal. I was able to see each dancer for only about half an hour. At a certain point, after seeing so many women with the same complaints, I realized that these dancers were barely subsisting on ibuprofen and diet soda, and they were suffering when on stage. Yet my only job for them was giving them spinal adjustments ("clicking" their backs) and wrapping their ankles and sending them away—to them, I was Clicky Vicky, the Wrapping Queen. This was soon after I'd developed my own understanding of Positive and Negative Feedback. I knew could do a lot more for my patients.

I started with the ballerinas. I'd analyze their entire health profile, going far beyond my official assignment of clicking and wrapping, but then I'd go back to the basics and say, "Yes, you've sprained this ankle, so you need to take a rest." I'd see the sense of relief on their faces, and when their defenses were down, I knew the time was right to dig a little deeper and help ease them into the Reflect phase, get them to consider where they were—and why.

Just as they were about to get up from the table, I'd stop them. "Now, let's talk about what's really going on: You're working like a robot, and you're taking painkillers to numb everything. You've already wrapped the ankle. You're covering up the problem. But actually, the *real* problem is that you're eating the wrong food and you're feeding your emotions. I'm guessing you're upset because your boyfriend left you or you broke up with someone. Am I right?"

At first they resisted. *Why is Clicky Vicky asking about my sex life?* But I persisted—I wanted to know more about the pain. And more important, I wanted *them* to know more about their pain—to ask questions of it, to seek wisdom in it. In my growth as a healer, I gained inspiration from Hippocrates: "A wise man should consider that health is the greatest of human blessings, and learn how by his own thought to derive benefit from his illnesses." *The body doesn't lie*—we just have to listen.

The more these conversations started to work, the more I could see my bigger purpose: I wasn't there just to wrap them and get them back up on stage. I was there to help them heal themselves.

These conversations blossomed into a deeper, more connected practice with my patients. These dancers were making major breakthroughs, coming to life-changing realizations: *Okay. I've sprained my ankle, and*

God is telling me to stop, rest, eat well. Even get a period. If I'm underweight and eating the wrong food, I'm eventually going to collapse. I have to take control of my life. Empower myself and think, "Hold on a second—I'm not weak, I'm strong. I'm a good professional dancer, but I need to respect other aspects of my life. I can't just be a good ballerina and not eat well and not meditate and not find time for me."

Throughout my years doing this work, I've seen many thousands of people at extraordinary moments in their lives: During labor. After falling off a horse. Before a world summit or a major performance. I've treated women who were having trouble getting pregnant. I've worked in children's clinics. And I've looked after many, many moms who have stopped looking after themselves.

I have seen repeatedly, during all these many experiences, that the trick to healing pain is taking the three steps to interrupt the Negative Feedback loop: *reflect* on the pain and how it got there; *release* the guilt, anger, and denial that are holding the pain inside you; and step out of your own shadow and *radiate* into your best life. Moving into the positive doesn't need to be an epic life makeover. Just one small choice, made consciously, can take you toward a better life. All you need is the recognition that it's time to start treating yourself as well as you treat everyone else—and a simple plan that can help you do just that.

Delicious food, centering meditations, healing movement, loving connections, rediscovered self-trust—all these help you liberate yourself from Negative Feedback and move into the positive. The Positive Feedback program isn't complicated or expensive—but it is powerful. If you're ready to make major changes, the program is here for you, ready to help in your transformation.

Listen, I know how hard you work. Throughout my life, and even now, I'm treating patients all day, often from 5:00 A.M. until 11:00 P.M. (or even, occasionally, until 2:00 A.M.!). I've always been this way, taking after my hardworking mom and her mother before her. We Greek ladies pour ourselves into work as an expression of love for our families—and I know we're not alone.

Regardless of the trappings of their lives, I find that most of my patients are women who are very busy, working, traveling. Dynamic women just starting their careers, or a bit further on, maybe with two or three kids. Passionate about what they do.

And all these women, no matter what their daily lives look like, are all on the path to learn the same thing: Healing can begin only when you have the courage to face the pain. In any pain scenario, you have to take a step back before you can take a step forward. No matter if the initial hurt was a simple childhood disappointment or a family scandal, the self-absorption that kept your mother at a distance or the fatal accident that took your brother from you—anything that's painful, no matter how traumatic, can be faced and released.

Every muscular ache/pain has a story; that neuromuscular memory started with a single moment. Pain constantly pulls us backward into the emotional and physical pit of our unhappiness. But we can stop the cycle and restore our more natural and positive balance. We're *meant* to be happy.

The Positive Feedback approach simply reinstates your innate inner strength, your natural ability to heal yourself, and your daily desire to be happy and whole. As I always say to my patients: It's not what happened to you that matters—it's what you do with that experience that will determine the quality of the rest of your life.

In the coming chapters, I will show you what an incredible positive force this resilience can be, and how it can transform pain into a powerful, healthy, pain-free radiance that lasts a lifetime.

How the Positive Feedback Program Works

When you give your full attention to your knee or your back or your head—whatever hurts—and drop the good/ bad, right/wrong story line and simply experience the pain directly for even a short time, then your ideas about the pain, and often the pain itself, will dissolve.

—Pema Chödrön

Dr. Andrew Taylor Still, the father of osteopathy, was ahead of his time. As far back as 1892, he believed that the human body was its own apothecary, that each body held all the chemicals and neurotransmitters needed to help a person fight disease and injury. Dr. Still believed that the body's ability to heal itself rested on the interplay between structure, function, and motion. Health started in the bones and was totally dependent on the open flow of blood in the body. Blockages equaled disease, so all healing began with an exam to find the blocks and a targeted release to get the blood flowing once again.

Here we are, over one hundred years later, and these ideas are still not mainstream—but we see them working every day. I see the validity of Dr. Still's approach when my patients are lying on the table and the acupuncture needles practically jump out of their shoulders or back; when they fall asleep on the table and are completely peaceful and relaxed; when they get up from the table and their whole demeanor is changed—the rosiness is back in their cheeks, and they feel alive again, at home in their body. They describe the feeling of energy moving back into their hands and feet, the sense that their mind seems clearer. They say things like, "I feel lighter," "My shoulders have dropped," "I feel more space in my body," "I feel grounded." "I'm ready to take on the world."

The same core mechanism that drives these osteopathic treatments powers the Positive Feedback program, because the Reflect * Release * Radiate sequence taps into the same biochemical responses in the body. Whether you have acupuncture, get a massage, or do your trigger points or dry brushing or Tibetan Rites, your body releases lymphatic fluids and your brain and central nervous system release natural painkillers, beta-endorphins. Just like osteopathic modalities, the Positive Feedback program also helps to soothe the hypothalamus—the part of the brain that links the nervous system to the endocrine system, the site of appetite and love and sexual energy and sleep—and quiet the panicked energy of the amygdala—the site of fear and stress and panic in the brain. Any of the program's activities will help you tone your parasympathetic nervous system and build your body's capacity to thoroughly relax and bounce back from stressful experiences.

That's the ultimate goal of each stage of the Reflect * Release * Radiate sequence: building your body's capacity. Both Positive and Negative Feedback start in a moment of stress, be it an acute injury or an exciting challenge. In Negative Feedback, rather than rise to meet the challenge, you shrink in defeat and get stuck in lethargy. You attach yourself to negative thoughts. You surround yourself with negative people. You either never, ever stop running—or you sink into inertia. (A body at rest stays at rest.)

Glucose builds up in your blood; plaque builds up in your brain and in your arteries; toxins build up in your liver. Your body responds to this systemic congestion with chronic inflammation, muscle atrophy, insulin resistance, and cognitive decline. Negative Feedback feeds on itself, keeping you trapped in pain.

But you have the power of choice. When faced with a challenge, if you rise to meet it, you become stronger going forward. Positive Feedback, as with negativity, also feeds on itself, so once you escape Negative Feedback, every second you spend in Positive Feedback strengthens this biological response: Your lymph nodes release accumulated waste. Your brain releases neurotoxins. Muscles build back up, insulin sensitivity increases again, and blood sugar drops. As blood sugar drops, chronic inflammation recedes and brain fog lifts. Circulation improves and blood pressure drops, putting a halt on cardiac risks. And all those improvements started with a simple choice—to meet the challenge, to feel the pain, and to move all the way through it.

A recent study of the Jewish Polish population that immigrated to Israel before and after World War II found that, compared with their contemporaries who'd been spared, men who'd been imprisoned during the Holocaust lived an average of ten to eighteen months longer than their peers who had not had that harrowing experience. Researchers believe that this "post-traumatic growth" is a perfect example of the Adaptive Response. Viktor Frankl, a psychiatrist who spent time in Auschwitz, and whose wife was killed in a different concentration camp, wrote *Man's Search for Meaning,* in which he argued that even in the most painful and horrifying situations, our lives and our suffering can have meaning. He wrote, "Between stimulus and response there is a space. In that space is our power to choose our response. In our response lies our growth and our freedom."

If people forced into the worst situation ever experienced by humankind can take a breath and choose their reaction—and choose to thrive despite the unspeakable horrors—we *all* have that power. All human greatness and resilience comes from this place of challenge and growth.

What doesn't kill me makes me stronger. Your Adaptive Response not only helps you heal from injury in the short term, it also improves your body's future healing potential. With a well-functioning Adaptive Response, you develop greater resistance to stress. Your endocrine system floods you with pleasure hormones, to congratulate you on a job well done. And while all these biochemical reactions to stress are going on, your neurological pathways are changing on a more permanent basis: Healthy choices become ingrained habits; healthy thoughts become empowering attitudes.

The biggest stumbling blocks that have thus far prevented you from entering Positive Feedback are these neural pathways. You must consciously and deliberately *choose* good habits at first. Making these choices can be a struggle sometimes—especially when you've been accumulating a ton of those unhealthy Band-Aids. But eventually, with enough physical and mental practice, they will no longer be choices; they will have become instincts.

To train yourself, rely on structure. Instead of seeing that structure as a jail that confines you, try to view it as a delicious and nourishing recipe for a better life. In order to ensure that your entire being is well cared for, I've organized all the self-care techniques of the Positive Feedback program into four categories, based on Dr. Still's work:

- Structure (focus on somatic symptoms via endorphin-boosting grooming, massage, self-healing trigger points, and other self-care)

- Function (focus on diet that includes nourishing, anti-inflammatory foods)

- Motion (focus on healing exercise that improves circulation and speeds lymphatic drainage)

- Emotion (focus on nurturing positive thoughts, feelings, and relationships)

You have to commit to implementing the Positive Feedback program in a systematic way, every day of your life. It almost doesn't matter what you focus on first, be it positive affirmations, healthy foods, a commitment to rest, or hydration and exercise—each of these habits strengthens your cells, your instincts, and your body's natural responses.

If you're just at the beginning of your healthy living journey, consider focusing on one category a day. As you progress and work toward four categories in a day, you'll see even more dramatic results. Following the program in a committed way ensures that your reactions will become more and more positive, because you'll develop habits and tools you can use to ensure that health will become your primary instinct.

Monica, a thirty-four-year-old marketing director and self-professed "perfection freak," describes her experience with the Positive Feedback program this way: "The thing I love about this program is that it takes away my perfectionism. I know I don't have to do everything perfectly. Every choice has the power to push me back into the positive." She knows that if she's been in Positive Feedback for a while, a glass of champagne or a late night isn't going to throw her back into Negative Feedback. But it does make her realize that each of those choices could be a trigger and could compound with others. She knows she could lose a lot of ground unless she sticks with the program. "But the best part is, I don't *want* to go negative," she says. "I know how good it feels to be in the positive, and how effortless it can be to stay there if I just keep focusing on that feeling, how wonderful and powerful I feel when I'm in the positive. Truly, I never want to leave again."

Once you see how the three steps work—the Reflect * Release * Radiate sequence—you can use those steps both as the structure for living and also as a decision-making technique. You'll learn to automatically apply the three steps to every challenge you face, every moment of pain you experience, every worry or moment of uncertainty you have—because you'll learn that these three steps, taken in this order, have the power to help you face any situation and come out the other end feeling stronger.

Let's take a quick look at how the program works. Then, in the three chapters of part 2, we'll consider the program in depth.

The Three Steps

Adaptive Response is the mechanism behind both vaccination and home-opathy: When exposed to a very small amount of a harmful antigen, your body not only repels the invading force, but also learns from the experience and grows stronger by developing antibodies that protect you from subsequent exposure. Going forward, anytime your body is exposed to that bacteria or virus again, these antibodies will prevent it from taking hold. In other words, your body has responded in an "adaptive" way—a healthy, positive, protective way.

Exposed to stresses every day—some good, some bad—your body tries to tap into this Adaptive Response constantly; in so doing, it's trying to grow stronger. If you pay attention to the structure, function, motion, *and* emotion of your body—if you feed your body well, take care of it, allow for ample activity and rest, face and express your emotions—then when you're exposed to a new stress, your body can make the most of it. Your body will turn that stress into a learning experience for itself, a "teachable moment," accessing your body's innate healing instinct.

REFLECT

"The unexamined life is not worth living." Socrates's timeless maxim reminds us that we need to constantly be looking at how we're moving through this world, keeping tabs on our thoughts and feelings, in order to give our experience any meaning at all. When you're in pain, you can be confounded by the effort it takes to simply get through the day. You might think, "I don't have time to deal with that pain: I have to get the kids to school, meet this work deadline, get Mom to the doctor's office." The list goes on and on. In a lifestyle of stalwart soldiering on, it takes strength to take a moment to stop and look at where you are, to *consciously* be in your body, to check in with your soul: *I am here. I am breathing. I feel anxious, but I can do this. What am I doing right now? Am I where I want to be?*

Developing the ability to check in with yourself may be the most powerful habit you learn in this program. Truly becoming in tune with yourself, your emotions, the feelings in your body as they are today is the first step toward any meaningful change. Simple awareness all by itself has the power to shift you into Positive Feedback, before you "do" anything else. All meditative practices start with awareness as the first step—in fact, it's the core of mindfulness meditation, one of most thoroughly researched and scientifically affirmed approaches.

Mindfulness trains us to be present in the moment. In focusing attention on the moment, you don't have to commit to a lifelong plan—or even a weeklong one. You just have to make a good choice *right now*. This skill immediately starts to transform your life by maximizing the beauty and stillness that can occur moment to moment. A nice walk. The feel of the sunshine. The taste of an apple. The smile of a friend. We learn to stop and appreciate these details through reflection. These are gifts from God—they feed our bodies and souls way more than any junk food or glass of wine ever could.

The Reflect phase, outlined in chapter 4, also helps to reverse our sympathetic nervous system overload. Our brains are so focused on the go-do-be culture of achievement and progress that we don't give our bodies the time they need to rest and recuperate. When we consciously make reflection part of our daily lives, we build up our parasympathetic nervous system. By focusing on awareness of the body, we develop a top-down orientation, from brain to body, that helps us relax thoroughly, ratchet down the heightened stress and anxiety, and decompress faster and more easily. Practiced regularly, reflection helps tone the PNS and reduce our blood pressure and stress hormones on a daily basis. This reduction in stress and anxiety then helps our bodies with the next two phases of the program—it helps us *release* toxins and eventually *radiate* our internal health to the world.

Rather than spending time wallowing in negative emotions, however, you should focus much of your reflection on reconnecting with your *physical* self. Most of us have spent years dissociating from our body. Now is the time to become reacquainted. In chapter 4, I introduce you to a body scan approach that will immediately bring you into the present moment with your body. This practice allows you to develop a "volume knob" for controlling your own brain's alpha rhythms. A study published in the *Frontiers of Human Neuroscience* found that meditation helps a person gain control of the alpha rhythms in the somatosensory cortex, a portion of the left frontal cortex that has a tremendous influence over negative thoughts and chronic pain.[1] Alpha waves are continually processing pain, so until you're able to control them, you may be unable to maintain attention on other tasks. But when you meditate on a consistent basis, you can improve your ability to focus and to regulate your emotional reactivity. By simultaneously tuning in to specific parts of your body, and tuning out negative thoughts and other aches or pains, you develop the coordination of your alpha rhythms and the ability to control your thinking at will. One study in the *Journal of Neuroscience* found that mindfulness meditation can lower pain levels by up to 57 percent.[2]

Several different activities (which I'll present in chapter 4) allow you to take a snapshot of where you are, capturing information to gain awareness of your body's current health status. These pieces of information can help you determine which areas you need to focus on during your Release stage. Many of my patients find that simply gathering the information is itself a therapeutic exercise. We don't give ourselves enough time to check in with our bodies and our minds on a regular basis. Giving ourselves permission to be "selfish" like this is a huge step forward for many of my patients—and I suspect it might be for you, too.

Being able to reflect will always help you—both by providing recognition of the way things truly are and by delivering you from denial. This practice also builds the mental and emotional foundation for the next elements of the program—the Release stage and the Radiate stage.

RELEASE

Release is the primary goal of many of my patients. They want to be released from pain, released from old hurts and traumas, released from pressure that keeps them from being happy. Many people come to osteopaths thinking that a click of the neck and a quick massage will do away with all the stress and anxieties that have built up over the past months (or years). But there is no amount of spinal manipulation that can equal your ability to release your own toxins. (For example, by this point in the program, you will have reestablished your commitment to a full night of quality rest, which has allowed your brain to release more toxins in seven days than I could ever do in seven treatments!)

Following guidelines given in chapter 5, you can learn a very simple but incredibly powerful technique for releasing self-healing trigger points. Using the same biomechanical mechanism at work in acupuncture, manipulation of these specific points will help you release your pain quickly. You can break the momentum of the Negative Feedback cycle long enough to give your body and brain a chance to let go and release in other ways as well. Freed from the most acute pain, you will be empowered with the space to explore ways that you can move your body and mind toward a healthier, more integrated, more fulfilling life. We'll talk through how you can forgive others for the pain they've caused you— and, more important, how you can forgive yourself and move on from ways that you've disappointed yourself. I'll walk you through the Release Meal Plan, a delicious cleansing regimen that taps into nature's most powerful anti-inflammatory foods to reverse the chronic inflammation that traps you in Negative Feedback.

Even though this is not specifically a weight loss plan, some people lose up to ten pounds during their initial Release week, and even more as they incorporate Release principles into their daily life. My client Reena found that steering clear of sugar for a week helped her break her addiction to sweet chai and introduced her to the cleansing wonders of nettle tea. Just that one change in her diet cut her chances of developing diabetes in half. Studies have shown that drinking large amounts of sugar-sweetened beverages can not only increase the risk of gaining weight but also of developing Type 2 diabetes, heart disease, and gout.[3] Over a couple of months, that one shift helped Reena remove fifteen pounds she'd been dragging around since graduate school six years earlier.

Psychological Antidotes

Rick Hanson, also the founder of the Wellspring Institute for Neuroscience and Contemplative Wisdom, has developed a series of psychological antidotes for psychologists and therapists to teach to patients (and use themselves!) when they are combating negative emotions and habits. These antidotes, listed in table 2, are great suggestions for anyone adopting the Positive Feedback program, because they give a focus point for affirmations and meditations.

When we spend too much time being ruled by our amygdala and our sympathetic nervous system, we remain locked in a negative outlook that perpetuates the triggering of stress hormones and clouds our perception of other people's intentions. Meditation, as noted earlier, offers multiple health benefits. Among those benefits: It has been found to decrease gray matter in the amygdala and increase gray matter in the hippocampus[4]—which is especially helpful in chronically nervous or stressed people, because severe stressful experiences can decrease hippocampal mass by up to 25 percent, depending on the severity of the experience.[5]

Table 2. **Psychological Antidotes to Common Emotional States**

IF YOU'RE EXPERIENCING ...	TRY FOCUSING YOUR MEDITATION ON ...
Weakness, helplessness, pessimism	Strength, efficacy
Alarm, anxiety	Safety, security
Resentment, anger	Compassion for oneself and others
Frustration, disappointment	Satisfaction, fulfillment
Sadness, discontent, "blues"	Gladness, gratitude
Rejection, feeling unseen or left out	Attunement, inclusion
Inadequacy, shame	Recognition, acknowledgment
Abandonment, feeling unloved or unlovable	Friendship, love

Adapted from Rick Hanson, "Mindfulness in Clinical Practice," paper delivered at the Northern California Psychiatric Society's Integrative Psychiatry Conference, Berkeley, CA, Sept. 10, 2011.

Are you concerned that a more controlled approach to food and cooking might leave you feeling miserable? Researchers at the University of Chicago suggest just the opposite. They found that the psychic effects of taking this kind of control can actually make you happier.[6] The fact that you no longer have to struggle with yourself about what you *should* do—now that you're automatically making the right choices—simplifies your life and makes you feel proud. We could call this the framework effect: Having an explicit program to hang on to and return to can quiet down the anxiety that extra choices provoke. I'll provide plenty of tips and suggestions in chapter 5 to help make the transition to anti-inflammatory foods satisfying and simple, and I'll offer meal plans and recipes in part 3.

I'll also guide you through some meditation and imagery that allows you to let go of the negative self-talk that plagues every person in Negative Feedback mode. These harsh words are what I think of as the "evil eye"—the negative specters of danger or worry that can cloud your psyche, even when you're not aware of them. Your continued meditation practice will start to increase the power of your brain's prefrontal cortex (PFC), the area of your brain that helps you stay on task and modulate your emotions. If you tend to be absentminded or short-tempered, it can be a sign that your prefrontal cortex isn't as healthy as it could be. Not only does this PFC weakness lead to emotional reactivity; in addition, by not helping to temper your sympathetic nervous system, your weak PFC may speed your aging. However, once you've been doing your Positive Feedback program for a week or two, you may find that you're becoming less emotionally reactive, less impulsive, and more focused. That's a sign that you've begun to take possession of that magic moment between stimulus and reaction—that moment that is the portal to the Adaptive Response. If you can choose to remain neutral and nonreactive in those split seconds, you'll more easily make the choices that keep you in the positive.

RADIATE

The Radiate phase involves discovering the full realization of who you were meant to be: your dreams, your passions. With your pain out of the way, important life goals begin to light you from within. Now that you've made it through the cleansing action of the vegetable-focused Release program, your palate is ready for more fruits, lean meats and goat's-milk yogurt (and other proteins), and occasional grains. Rather than start a vigorous exercise program just for vanity's sake, one that might throw you back into an inflammatory state, work on developing an individualized fitness approach that helps strengthen your ever-broadening sense of connection with the world.

Maybe you'll take up overnight backpacking; maybe you'll schedule a long-distance biking trip; maybe you'll sign up for a trip to Machu Picchu or a 5K run to benefit a charity you feel strongly about. No matter what kind of exercise you select, you'll reap the benefits of exercise's ability to increase your body's supply of brain-derived neurotrophic factor (BDNF). This miracle protein not only creates new brain cells and increases brain volume but also helps regulate blood sugar and encourage cardiovascular health, particularly by helping to further strengthen your parasympathetic nervous system.[7]

Once you get to the Radiate stage, you will spend much more of your time consciously basking in the beauty of your life, sinking deep into it. Training yourself to really key into the experience will help to counteract any negative conditioning you've experienced. Drawing on the skills you developed in the Reflect stage, you'll be mindful of shifts in your mood and take care to thoroughly drench yourself in the neurochemical bliss that's triggered by happy moments. The neurotransmitters that are released with success and happiness—endorphins, dopamine, serotonin, norepinephrine, and acetylcholine—will help you develop the inner strength, self-confidence, resilience, and determination to go out and achieve other goals.

As you become more mindful of how you feel, you develop your ability for meta-cognition—in other words, for thinking about how you think. You're able to be reflective and self-aware in every moment, without it feeling awkward or navel-gazey. True self-awareness, no longer being divorced from your feelings, will allow you to feel and experience new pain right away, before it can take root in your body. You will start to

A Positive Feedback Profile

Jennifer, a thirty-five-year-old woman, came to me complaining of lower back pain. Immediately it was clear that she was stuck in the negative. She had been jumping from relationship to relationship, always hoping for the right guy to marry, but having no luck. The morning she came to see me, she had developed an itchy rash all over her body.

"Do you think my body is allergic to Steve?" she asked, referring to her most recent sexual partner. As she told me about this particular womanizer, a man who apparently just wanted to drink and take drugs, I realized how toxic he was for her. *The body doesn't lie.*

Jennifer was a beautiful, intelligent woman, but she wasn't working or using her talents in a productive way. She told me that she'd always been close to her older sister, Suzanne. Now, though, she felt left out of her sister's life. Suzanne had kids and a thriving career, and Jennifer felt like she had nothing. "My sister tells me I just have to grow up, cleanse my system, and move ahead."

As we talked, the full picture began to emerge—and all Jennifer's concerns found themselves centered on her lower back pain (see table 3). We walked through the Reflect exercises, and discussed how she would create her Body Timeline, Body Family Tree, and Time Audit. We discussed the fact that lower back pain was often a signal of someone or something going wrong in a person's life. I advised her to follow the full Positive Feedback program for three weeks, and asked her to focus on her relationship with Suzanne. I knew that Jennifer needed to heal that connection in order to help herself make forward progress as well.

Take a look in table 4 at the specific tasks we devised for her—and notice how each phase helped her move out of her "stuckness" and into the next phase.

You can see from Jennifer's plan that she didn't incorporate every single exercise from the Positive Feedback program. What she did was select the exercises or changes that she believed would have the greatest impact on her life, and she followed through on those. The Positive Feedback plan helped her create the structure she needed to give her safe passage out of the woods of her pain and into the promise of one less loser lover, two adoring nieces, and a more fulfilling, more mature future.

Table 3. **A Symptom-Source Case Study**

SITE OF JENNIFER'S PAIN	PHYSICAL SYMPTOMS	EMOTIONAL SOURCE
T1, T2 (thoracic spine) L2, L3 (lumbar spine)	Shortness of breath, panic attacks, depression, low energy, lower back pain, insomnia	Fear of life, loss of power, anger, blocked sexual chakra

Table 4. **An Individualized Positive Feedback Prescription**

JENNIFER'S POSITIVE FEEDBACK PRESCRIPTION	JENNIFER'S REPORT
Need to REFLECT: Using the Body Timeline, Family Tree, and Time Audit, acknowledge your fears and recognize the memory of pain from your past. Create a new visualization and meditation to remind yourself that you're not a victim and your trauma is not, nor has it ever been, a case of life and death.	"As I reflected using these tools, I realized that I'm afraid I'm no longer my sister's top priority—but I completely understand, too. Her family needs her; I need to focus on healing myself instead of waiting for her to rescue me. I need to get out of my bad relationship and take a break from men for a while so I can focus on myself."
Need to RELEASE: Expand your Morning Glory routine to include dry brushing and scrub several layers of calloused skin off your feet; then get a pedicure to show them off! Swap repeated sweet coffees and diet sodas for a few liters of lemon water per day, to help rehydrate long-parched tissues and sweep out any toxins lingering in the gut. Create a meditation to release anger and resentment toward Suzanne.	"I realized that I had to release my toxic food habits—no more diet soda and white pasta for me—and the contrast once I got started was shocking. As I included more fish and vegetables in my diet, my energy level soared; I no longer felt like a weeping pile of aimless mush in the afternoon. I stayed clear-headed without all the coffee and soda, and slept better than I had in years."

JENNIFER'S POSITIVE FEEDBACK PRESCRIPTION	JENNIFER'S REPORT
Need to RADIATE: Choose a "passion project," something that will help you feel connected to the community and be of service to others. Learn to cook two exotic meals just for yourself!	"I realized that, because of my dependence on Suzanne, I'd been resenting her kids. I resolved to have a better relationship with them. In my new role as Auntie Cici, I researched different day trips for us to do (which also gave Suzanne some much-needed time alone). The kids and I created a ritual of visiting a restaurant and then trying to recreate our favorite meal together at home the next day. I also started waking up early to do yoga or go walking along the beach at sunrise—my daily reminder to radiate!"

see what patterns make your body and your mind feel stronger, cleaner, healthier—and which ones leave you feeling trapped in the negative. You'll be living in the positive and thriving.

You'll also become more compassionate to the suffering of others, a proven remedy for loneliness and isolation. One Harvard study found that eight weeks of meditation training was all it took for people to become 35 percent more compassionate to the suffering of others.[8] By getting out of your own way and reawakening to the beauty in the world, you'll be able to find your way out of the fog of negativity faster and more easily. You'll have built a map for yourself, a way out of the woods of your pain.

Your newfound compassion and honesty with yourself will allow you to form true connections with others, and those connections themselves can be therapeutic.

Finally, the master skill that you'll develop in the Radiate phase is the strength to be courageous about taking risks in your own life, to—as author Susan Jeffers puts it—"feel the fear and do it anyway."[9] Research has proven, both in animal studies and with humans, that when we're faced with fear, if we can steel our resolve and just "get on with it," we can break down conditioned responses that would otherwise hold us back. Conquering our fears helps us develop a sense of "agency" that translates into other fields. Simply put, we have the ability to survive and even thrive, no matter what occurs.

Yes, this is my ultimate dream: You will let go of any remaining fears that have held you back and, armed with your own confidence and your ability to grit your teeth through your anxiety, you will find that there's nothing you can't do. You will feel stronger and more alive, and you will radiate strength and beauty.

Preparing to Start the Positive Feedback Program

No matter what kind of pain you're in right now, when you start the Positive Feedback plan, you'll be able to restore your innate Adaptive Response, rebuild your body's foundation, and claim the life you were always meant to live. All it takes is the determination to spend a little bit of time on yourself each day. This small commitment to focus on your own self-care can help you learn to nurture and protect your inner self.

Even if you get off track, Positive Feedback is always there for you. At any time, and every time. The program will never be "too hard"— Positive Feedback begins the very moment you do the Morning Glory ritual. Once you get into that positive cycle, the momentum of the Reflect * Release * Radiate sequence has a way of carrying you to the next stage of health, and the next, and the next. So let's get started on that transformation already!

I encourage you to read all the way through the next three chapters to get a good sense of what's to come. And although you can follow most of the program using supplies already available around your house, you may need to gather some additional materials (such as a bag of lemons for your daily lemon water, or a dry brush to use in your Morning Glory routine starting in the Release phase). In appendix C, I've also shared a shopping list of foods for the Release week. Wait until the day before you start that phase to shop for those foods, so you can have your produce at its peak of freshness.

I would also suggest that you choose a notebook or small three-ring binder to keep with you throughout the program, to capture your observations during your Reflect exercises (Body Timeline, Body Family Tree, Time Audit, etc.) and to collect notes about foods to avoid or new products you'd like to try. (In appendix B, you'll find a collection of foods and personal care products that I love and try to use every day.) Some people find it helpful to copy into a notebook the words of meditations that they find particularly meaningful or helpful. Alternatively, you could record them with your phone or a handheld recorder and play them for yourself until you remember them by heart.

Please note: I heartily encourage you to improvise. If the italicized words in any meditation don't work for you, create your own. You can use your notebook to write out the scripts for your own personal meditations and visualizations to help you stay consistent from one week to the next. Just the act of writing down a meditation will be therapeutic on its own. Personally, I like to take five minutes at the end of every day to write a simple paragraph in my journal, to remind me of the beautiful things that happened that day. You might consider using your Positive Feedback notebook for that purpose as well, so you can look back and trace how your state of mind shifts while you're following the three steps.

Over the next three weeks, this progressive system of self-care strategies and rituals will help you *reflect* on your life, *release* what's polluting you and causing you pain, and *radiate* into a more beautiful and satisfying way of living. The structure of this plan will help you make immediate, pain-relieving changes to your self-talk, eating habits, exercise regimen, and morning routine. Some of these changes will be easy to implement; some will be more challenging. I firmly believe that you will get out of this program every ounce of work you put into it.

Your new life is right around the corner. Let's see what's in store for you in the first week of the Positive Feedback program: the Reflect phase.

PART TWO

The Positive Feedback Program

Week 1: Reflect

Life can only be understood backwards;
but it must be lived forwards.

—Søren Kierkegaard

W hen I was a young girl, my mother counseled me to start every morning by looking in the mirror. "Take a good look at yourself, Vicky. Look at how beautiful you are. See the things you love. And also see the things you'd like to change," she'd say. "Now, make a plan to change them."

In order to get back into Positive Feedback, you must understand all the aspects of your health and your environment that are putting stress on your body. Once you have a full understanding of these factors, you can move into the Release phase and start to let them go.

The main task of your Reflect time is to become mindful—to truly *feel* your pain—because pain is the message, the teacher. Pain tells you where you need to focus. Your goal during reflection is to increase awareness, become rooted in your body once again. Many people in pain do everything they can to get out of their body—to get away from that pain. *You* are going to face it; now, during the Reflect week, you're going to deliberately set aside time to be brave, pull back the curtain of denial, and take a good look at everything you're doing in and to your body—and your mind.

The only way you can move forward is if you see and experience and acknowledge the pain—only then can you release it. The following are exercises and techniques that let you step back, look at your life, and give you the whole picture.

Laying the Foundation

The foundation of the Positive Feedback program consists of two daily practices:

- Get seven to eight hours of quality sleep

- Carry out the Morning Glory ritual

These practices will help put you in a new mind-set. In fact, if you're like most of my patients who shortchange themselves on sleep and self-care, I promise that if you do just these two things, your life will radically improve in just a few days.

SUFFICIENT QUALITY SLEEP

Sleep is the most regenerative, restorative, automatic biological process humans experience—so why on earth do we skimp? Many people pretend they can get by on five or six hours a night, but nothing could be further from the truth. We need at least seven hours of solid sleep a night in order to stay out of sleep deficit.

Chronic sleep deprivation leads to horrible consequences: memory loss (and eventual brain damage), excess pounds, increased insulin, increased hunger and stress hormone levels, increased blood pressure, and decreased immunity. Without enough high-quality sleep, your body doesn't have time to rest and regenerate; as a result, your tissues age literally overnight.

On the upside, improving sleep may nudge you out of Negative Feedback all by itself: A study of patients with chronic sleep deficits found that just one month of improved sleep significantly reduced their levels of tumor necrosis factor and C-reactive protein, both markers for systemic inflammation.[1] Recent research from the University of Rochester found that our brains have a so-called glymphatic system—a drainage system akin to our lymphatic system, organized by neurons called glial cells, that helps the brain release toxins during sleep. These scientists found that while we sleep, this glymphatic system is ten times more active than when we are awake, and the pathways in our brain expand by a staggering *60 percent,* allowing our cerebrospinal fluid to wash away the brain's amyloid plaques that are believed to cause Alzheimer's. The restorative quality of sleep may be the result of this enhanced removal of potentially neurotoxic wastes that accumulate in our nervous system during our waking hours.[2] I believe this is the same mechanism that makes cranial sacral therapy such a powerful healing modality—I swear my patients look ten years younger afterward! And this research shows you have access to this powerful anti-aging mechanism in your own bed, every single night.

I want you to vigilantly protect your sleep as you would that of your own baby or youngster. You would never prevent a tired child from sleeping, after all. (In fact, a mother would probably do just about anything to make sure her child got the recommended ten to twelve hours—if only to stave off whining the next day!)

Some self-care strategies take work to implement. Sleep isn't one of them. I know you already sleep like a champ at least sometimes! All I'm asking is for you to surrender a little more easily, a little earlier, and a little more deeply. Sleep should *not* be seen as a luxury. And, really, what are you doing that's more important? Checking social media? Head-bobbing your way through Jimmy Kimmel?

Stress, emotional upset, and physical aches and pains all can lead to sleep struggles. Whether you have sleep issues or not, I urge you to try a few of these tips that I share with my patients to ensure a deep, restful seven to eight hours of sleep:

- Drink lots of water during the day, but stop three hours before bed to avoid getting up to use the toilet. Then drink one cup of caffeine-free chamomile tea about an hour before lights out.

- Turn off the heat at night and leave the window very slightly open. Normally, your body cools down at night and warms up again as a signal for awakening. Insomnia can be caused by internal heat or inflammation.

- If you don't get to bed on time, try to sleep in as long as you can! (But don't make a habit of it—shoot to get to bed by ten, but certainly before midnight, at the latest.) And definitely schedule a power nap—no more than twenty-five minutes, or you'll fall into deep sleep and disrupt your sleep for the coming night.

- If you find that you enjoy the Tibetan Rites in your Morning Glory routine, consider adding them to your evening routine as well, either after work, just before dinner, or before bath time. Similarly, a ten- to fifteen minute meditation works as a sleep aid: My patients who practice evening meditation for two weeks or so generally start forgetting to take their sleeping pills.

- Take a relaxing bath with Epsom salts and add some drops of frankincense or sandalwood oil to the water. Light candles and/or incense and make a peaceful, calming environment where you can clear your mind, let go of negative thoughts and stress, reflect on your day, and forgive and be grateful.

- Leave all electronics out of the bedroom—no iPads or iPhones, please. Your charging station should be elsewhere in the house, such as the bathroom or kitchen. One exception: the Jawbone UP, or similar device, can help you track your hours of sleep (see Resources for information).

- If you've had long-standing insomnia, get a jump on a couple of dietary changes. (If you sleep reasonably well already, simply follow the dietary suggestions noted in the "Positive Function" section later in this chapter; you'll make more radical dietary changes in the Release stage.) Avoid eating sugar, spices, and especially spicy food at night, as the heat from spice may wake you up between 3:00 and 5:00 A.M. No diet soda, either. And eat a light dinner. No heavy meals of beef or lamb; if you must have meat, try just a light, easy-to-digest fish meal. My patients who eat salad for dinner find that they have improved sleep. If you go that route, be sure to add olive oil, lemon, and walnuts—but no balsamic vinegar (high in sugar).

- Drink no more than one coffee after breakfast and, if you must, one last coffee after lunch, but before three thirty at the latest (organic coffee only).

- If you're *really* having trouble sleeping, try Valerian root capsules (*Valeriana officinalis* combined with *Humulus lupulus,* or hops fruit). Follow package instructions for recommended dosages, and take the medication thirty minutes before sleep.

Truly the best sleep aids I've found? Laugh a lot, relax, and have sex—these are keys to longevity *and* sleep.

THE MORNING GLORY RITUAL

I do this ritual every single morning to get grounded and ready for my day. If your system has been chaotic and out of alignment, if you've been out of your body, so to speak, if your mind has been clouded, or if it's simply been a while since you've truly felt in touch with yourself inside your skin, this routine is just the thing to bring you back into the positive. Several studies have found that rituals themselves—regardless of what they are or the purpose they serve!—help you feel more in control and in the moment; and this effect endures even when you're at your most depressed.[3]

The Morning Glory ritual is actually a mini-version of the entire program: You reflect, release, and radiate, all within twenty to thirty minutes (depending on where you are in the program). Do this basic routine every single morning. (During the next two stages of the Positive Feedback program, you will intensify the experience with subtle adjustments that help to deepen the Release and Radiate aspects of the ritual.)

Before your first Morning Glory ritual, find (or clear) a space in your house that's just for you—a comfortable, clean, quiet area where you can do your meditation and light exercises. Have handy a yoga mat or blanket

Reflect-Week Morning Glory Ritual at a Glance

- Warm water with lemon
- Tibetan Rites of Rejuvenation exercises
- Breathing exercise
- Daily reflection
- Shower
- Self-massage with oil
- Morning meditation (focused on gratitude, acceptance)

or towel (or even something special like a sarong from a tropical voyage) that you can lie on. Consider turning part of this area into a small altar with candles or incense, a healthy plant (for extra oxygen), a photograph of someone you love, and perhaps some beautiful fabrics and cushions or rose quartz (a symbol of love and protection). Make this sacred space warm and lovely. You will return to it every day for your Morning Glory ritual, as well as for the positive affirmation and meditation breaks you take throughout your day. (Please note that this space can be portable: You can take your sarong and rose quartz with you, for example, and use them to recreate the space in any break room, locker room, or hotel room.) The key is to make all the elements you use feel and look beautiful—to help reflect your own beauty back to you.

Make time for the Morning Glory ritual by waking up twenty minutes earlier than you have been—before work or before your kids are awake—so you can find some *me* time and not mummy/work/crazy time. Set your alarm to chime a bell or other tone that's not jarring. If you live in a semiprivate neighborhood, consider leaving your shades open to allow the sun's light to wake you. (Your body's whole circadian clock can be realigned by waking to natural light.) Ideally, you'll get to a place where your body doesn't need an alarm to wake up.

Go to the kitchen and start your day with a glass of lukewarm filtered water with the juice of half a lemon. Lemon is a marvel. It helps flush out toxins in the gastrointestinal tract, helps strengthen the immune system, contains cortisol-lowering vitamin C, and contains enzymes that support the regeneration of the liver, our main detoxifying and fat-burning organ. Drink the entire glass as you look out the window at the dawn of a new day. Say quietly or silently,

> I am grateful for this day. I am grateful for my life, my body,
> my family, my love [whomever you love]. I am eager to see what
> my day holds.

Go to your quiet space and do the five Tibetan Rites of Rejuvenation exercises to clear your mind. This method is powerful enough to wake up your circulation, yet gentle enough to help you slowly regain fitness if you're in pain.

Thanks to my mother's wonderful influence, I've been doing this series of exercises since I was a little girl. The Tibetan Rites are a sequence of five poses believed to be several thousand years old that have been called "a fountain of youth." First introduced to the West in 1939 in a quirky book called *The Eye of Revelation* by Peter Kelder, the Tibetan Rites are being embraced more and more as a rejuvenating, simple, portable, cost-free exercise program that can keep your chakras open (Kelder called them "vortexes"), your circulation flowing, your balance fine-tuned, and your muscles fit and strong until well into your golden years. (You'll notice, in figures 4 through 8, that several of the poses are very similar to yoga!) Please note: Throughout each of the exercises, please breathe only through your nose with your mouth closed. "Pump" your breath through your nostrils. If you're doing it correctly, your breath will be loud—don't be embarrassed! This is the way it should sound. The sound of your breath will also help your concentration.

No matter where I am in the world, I do this sequence every single day, without fail; it is my touchstone, my center. Sometimes, when I need an extra boost, I'll even do it twice a day. I do twenty-one repetitions of each pose, which the original text stated was the optimum number. Start slow, with increments of three repetitions, and work up to twenty-one. In between each exercise, lie on the floor, and take three deep breaths, in and out through your nose.

The Five Tibetan Rites of Rejuvenation Exercises

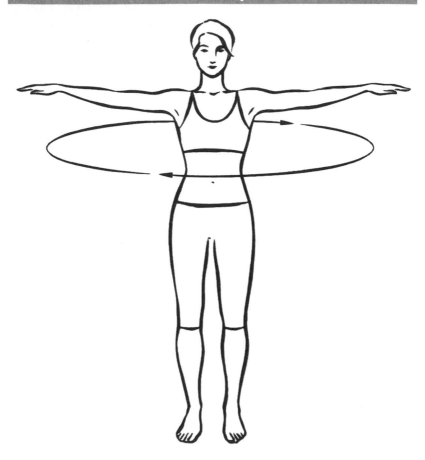

Rite No. 1   Stand tall and long, as if you have a string from the top of your head to the ceiling, with your arms outstretched. Concentrate on stretching your middle finger as far as possible. Keep your shoulders back and down, relax your jaw, and keep your tummy pulled in. Keep your eyes open and select a point on the wall to orient yourself and to help you count. Turn from left to right (clockwise), pivoting around your right foot, taking small, rapid steps, inhaling and exhaling deeply as you spin. Most adults can spin only about six times before they become dizzy. If you become dizzy, please stop, bring your hands together, interlace your fingers, and bring your hands to your heart. Stare at your thumbs and breathe deeply until the dizziness passes. Then you can start again. Start with three repetitions and by the end of Radiate, work up to twenty-one.

When you are done with your repetitions, lie flat on the floor, and take three deep breaths through your nose.

The Five Tibetan Rites of Rejuvenation Exercises

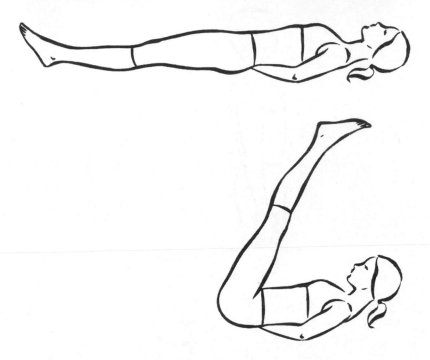

Rite No. 2   From this position, place your hands underneath your lower back and upper buttocks. Fingers should be kept close together with the fingertips of each hand turned slightly toward those of the other hand. Index finger should meet index finger, and thumb should meet thumb, to form a little triangle to cushion and protect the spine under the sacrum/coccyx. Breathe in and hold it, and raise your neck gently, pushing down slightly on your elbows to protect your neck. Then raise your feet until your legs are straight up, with big toe against big toe. If possible, let your feet extend back a bit over the body, toward the head, but don't let your legs bend. Then slowly lower your feet to the floor and allow the muscles to relax. Finally, slowly let go of your neck and breathe out. (This entire motion should happen with one breath.) Repeat the entire sequence again, working up to twenty-one times.

When you are done with your repetitions, lie flat on the floor, and take three deep breaths through your nose.

The Five Tibetan Rites of Rejuvenation Exercises

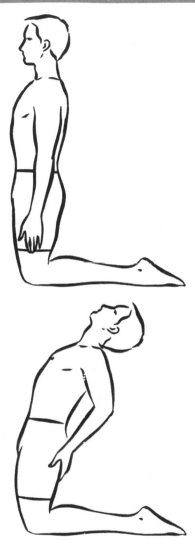

Rite No. 3   Kneel down on the floor and place your hands on the back of your thighs (or, if you have lower back pain, place your palms on your lower back). Exhale and lean your head forward until your chin rests on your chest. Keeping your chin tucked, inhale and lean backward until you feel the stretch in your thighs. Hold your tummy in and clench your buttocks, for extra support. Repeat, inhaling as you arch the spine and exhaling as you straighten.

When you are done with your repetitions, lie flat on the floor, and take three deep breaths through your nose.

The Five Tibetan Rites of Rejuvenation Exercises

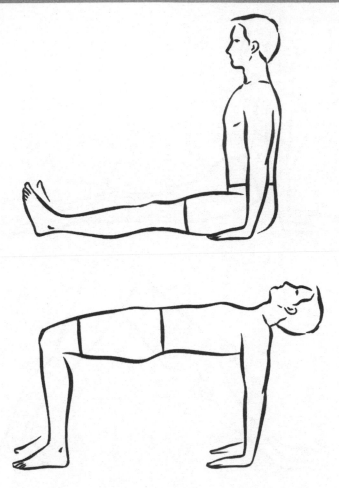

Rite No. 4   Move into a sitting position on the floor with your feet stretched out in front of you. Flex your feet. Place your hands on the floor next to your hips. Now tuck your chin to your chest. Breathe in and raise your body and bend your knees so that the legs, from the knees down, are practically vertical, like a table. The arms, too, will be straight up and down, while the body, from the shoulders to the knees, will be horizontal. Allow your head to gently drop back as far as it will go. Breathe out and return to a sitting position, relax for a moment, and then repeat.

When you are done with your repetitions, lie flat on the floor, and take three deep breaths through your nose.

The Five Tibetan Rites of Rejuvenation Exercises

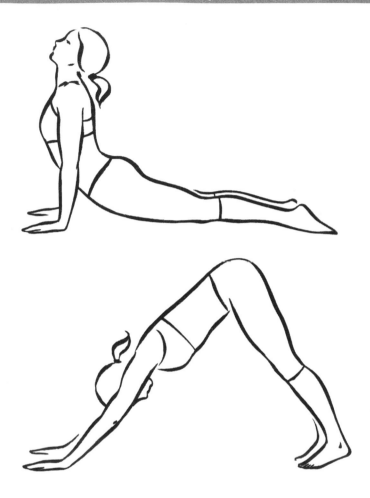

Rite No. 5   From a kneeling position, place your hands on the floor about two feet apart and stretch your legs out to the rear, with the feet about two feet apart. Stretch your fingers out wide, and then, bearing your weight on arms and toes, breathe out and allow the body to sag down and bring the head up, pulling it back as far as possible without hyperextending. Then breathe in and push the hips up as far as they will go; at the same time, bring your chin toward your chest. Draw your belly button in toward your spine. Repeat, breathing in as you raise the body and exhale fully as you lower the body.

When you've completed the Tibetan Rites, finish by lying on your back with your knees bent, close your eyes, and do this brief breathing exercise: Place your left hand on your heart and your right hand on your tummy. Take a deep breath, inhaling and exhaling from your nose only. Allow your stomach to expand on the inhale and retract on the exhale. (Make sure that you reach the "bottom" of your lungs, then exhale—that triggers a relaxing parasympathetic nervous system reflex.) Repeat three times.

Before showering but after you take your clothes off, face yourself in the mirror: It's time for your daily reflection. Many of my patients resist doing this simple act—they find themselves pointing out all the things they don't like. Instead of doing that, instead of judging yourself at all—good or bad—just really *look*.

See your face. See your neck, your shoulders, your chest. Look directly at your belly. Simply look—do not judge and do not label, but do not look away.

Every day, spend a full minute (it feels longer than it is) just looking at yourself. This exercise will help bring you back into your body, back into awareness of your physical being. Tell yourself:

> I am starting to take control of my body, my mind, and my
> emotions. I am starting to clean myself up. I am the power and
> authority. I am taking control of my body; I am taking control
> of my life, my fears, my insecurities, and any guilty feelings that
> create pain in my life.

Remember that you can always substitute language that makes you feel more comfortable, but it has to be positive and supportive.

Now it's time for your shower. Make the water warm to comfortably hot. As you step in, notice the water washing over your skin. Notice the way the shower cascades over your scalp. Feel the warmth seeping into your skin, your bones. Notice the steam rising up around you, the rhythm of the droplets hitting the tiles, creating a soothing din. For now, in this initial week, wash your hair and body as you normally would. We'll add to this process in the Release stage. Finish with a nice cold rinse.

Dry your body with a thick towel. (Splurge on a hotel-type towel and hoard it in your bathroom—no sharing with your spouse or your kids!) Now massage your body, from fingertips to toes, with a scented oil or moisturizer. Use "happy" oils—a couple drops of lemon, grapefruit, or peppermint essential oil added to unscented massage oil or sweet almond, grapeseed, or coconut oil will make you more awake, alert, and aware. Notice the way your hand glides over your skin. Notice the way your body feels smoother and more limber after your shower—fresh, cold, and awake—and how your skin drinks in the oil to prolong the smoothness.

End your Morning Glory routine with a morning meditation that sets the tone for your day. Move to your sacred space and sit or lie down. (Or, if you prefer, you may remain standing.) Try to clear your mind and start your day on a positive, relaxed note. Placing your left hand to your heart area and your right hand on your tummy, speak aloud to yourself (or to God or the universe or any power greater than yourself):

> I am grateful for all that I have. I love my body. I give myself the
> gift of forgiveness, and I am free. I allow joy and sweetness in
> my life. I love my life. I love how I feel today.

Repeat this meditation three times. Important: Please say these words (or equally positive words). You're training your mind to change the way you view yourself and your life. Your thoughts create your reality.

Take a deep cleansing breath, in through the nose, out through the mouth. Now you're ready to start your day.

As I mentioned, the Morning Glory ritual is a mini-program that comprises all three components. This daily routine allows you to head into your day ready and armed for anything that comes your way. Combined with your commitment to seven or eight hours of quality sleep, your Morning Glory ritual is the foundation that stops the negative and helps find and retain the positive. Protect this time as sacred; promise yourself that even if the rest of your life gets nuts, you'll always go back to these two foundational practices. They'll keep you on the right path.

Now let's dig in a bit deeper into the meat of the first step of the program. As I mentioned in chapter 3, each of the stages of the Positive Feedback program is organized into four categories: structure (focus on somatic symptoms), function (focus on diet), motion (focus on exercise), and emotion (focus on thoughts, feelings, and relationships). We'll start with establishing Positive Structure.

Positive Structure

The Positive Feedback program contains several exercises that will help you achieve positive structure. The first is to make a Body Map.

BODY MAP

When people come into my office, many can't articulate in words where they feel the pain; it's easier for them to show me in pictures. This works well for me, because it's how I keep records in their charts. This approach will help you, too.

Examine the paired diagrams in figure 9. (These diagrams are also available at www.elixirliving.com) Make several photocopies of the diagrams so that you can trace your progress over time. Start by making notations near the parts of your body where you feel pain or discomfort. Just make small notes in the margins: "Burning in my right shoulder blade." "Dull ache in my lower back." "Tightness in my neck muscles."

After you complete your first full cycle of the Positive Feedback program, you will take out a clean page and record your feelings again. Are there any differences? This comparison will give you valuable insight into your progress. Simply making the notes is itself a form of progress, however, because in doing so you begin to pay greater attention to your physical being. Repeat this evaluation often so that you stay connected with your body; then you'll be able not only to reflect upon and appreciate the progress you're making, but also to quickly notice subtle shifts in ongoing issues *before* you fall into Negative Feedback. You'll also have a wealth

Figure 9. **Body Map Template**

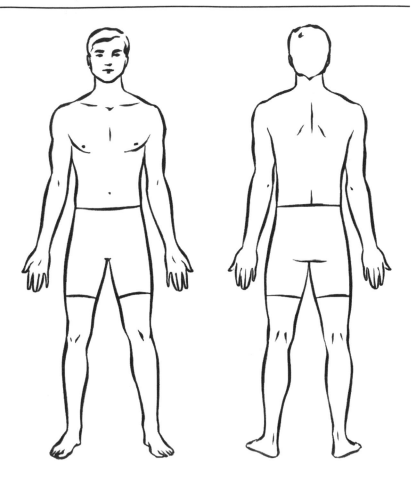

of information to share with your doctor or other health practitioner. Finally, many people with chronic pain have found that keeping a diary of symptoms can help them feel more in control.

BODY FAMILY TREE

Often, I ask my patients about their family history of cancer, heart disease, thyroid conditions, or depression, and they have no idea. They might know about their dad's high cholesterol or their mom's colonoscopy scare—but beyond those isolated instances, they really don't have a clue about their genetic history.

Your Body Family Tree may take you some time to create, but it will be worth it. (See figure 10 for a sample.) You'll learn a great deal about yourself and your unique genetic makeup. Talk to your siblings, mother, and father about their health experiences, and get as much information as you can about your grandparents (and even great-grandparents!). While you're listening to family stories, you'll likely gain clarity about the origins of some of your own struggles and vulnerabilities. This powerful tool will help you better understand your personal history and also can strengthen your compassion for your family members. This exercise is not meant to scare you—it's about acknowledging your family history and stopping negative patterns.

Another purpose that your Body Family Tree serves is as a record. Many of my patients will say to me something like, "I think Mom told me that she had a cyst once," but they can't remember where it was located, when it was discovered, or how it was removed. (This information sits in the back of your brain, creating unconscious worry.) Questions are even more likely with older relatives: "I think my mom's grandmother had breast cancer, but I don't know any details. I never even met her." Writing down that sort of information in one place will help you reflect on your history while holding on to it for the future. You can even bring a copy with you to any doctor's appointment. You may start to see patterns, such as all the women in your family live into their nineties and tend to have huge families—and you can be grateful for strong longevity or fertility genes. Or you may finally realize that six of your close relatives have diabetes, and you've developed a little belly and skinny legs—the family tree may help you realize that you should really get tested for pre-diabetes or insulin resistance. Prevention is better than cure!

One of my patients had struggled with feelings of low self-esteem and seasonal depression for years. Jackie could see that she wasn't alone: Her mom was incredibly anxious, her sister seemed angry all the time for no reason, and her father was cold and distant. Yet depression was a taboo

Figure 10. **Sample of Your Body's Family Tree**

CONDITION	YOU	MOM	DAD
Autoimmune/Allergies: Celiac, lupus, rheumatoid arthritis, MS, Type 1 diabetes, asthma, allergies, etc.			
Behavioral Health: Addiction, anxiety, depression, self-harm, anorexia, bulimia, etc.	Anxiety	Anxiety	
Cancer: Breast, cervical, lung, prostate, skin, uterine, etc.	Cervical	Cervical	
Cardiovascular: Stroke, heart attack, high blood pressure, high cholesterol, etc.		High blood pressure, high cholesterol	High blood pressure, high cholesterol, stroke
Digestive: Colitis, acid reflux, Crohn's, irritable bowel syndrome			
Endocrine: Type 2 diabetes, Cushing's, thyroid, etc.			
Musculoskeletal: Broken bones, osteoporosis, arthritis, bone spurs, etc.	Broken bone	Arthritis	
Neurological: Autism, Alzheimer's, ADHD, schizophrenia, bipolar, etc.	Anxiety, ADHD	Anxiety	Asperger's
Reproductive: Fertility problems (male or female), PMS, PMDD, early menopause, etc.		Early menopause	

SIBLINGS	GRAND-MOTHERS	GRAND-FATHERS	AUNTS OR UNCLES	DISTANT RELATIVES
Addiction	Anxiety		Anxiety	Anxiety, addiction
	Uterine	Leukemia	Breast, prostate	
	High blood pressure, high cholesterol	High blood pressure, high cholesterol, stroke	High blood pressure, high cholesterol, heart attack	
Acid reflux				
Broken bone				
Anxiety, ADHD	Alzheimer's	Bipolar	Alzheimer's	Schizophrenia
PMDD				

subject in her house growing up. As a teenager, she yearned to get some help, to talk to a therapist—anything. But she got the message loud and clear that sharing fears or talking about mental health was just not something her family did—much easier to point at the other person and say, "What's wrong with you?"

Jackie started drinking, smoking cigarettes, and smoking pot as a teenager, to escape her feelings of anxiety, and these habits carried through her twenties. By the time Jackie came to me in her early thirties, she'd started having panic attacks. Her neck had seized up and she was complaining of heart palpitations. I sent her home with a packet of Positive Feedback materials and the name of a good therapist. I told her to come back for another appointment and be prepared to discuss her family history.

When she returned, I could see that some weight had already been lifted. "I'd never asked my mom about our family medical history before," she said. "I can't believe how much I learned about myself!" Turns out, when Jackie sat down to complete the Body Family Tree, she saw very clearly that her family history was rife with mental health issues. All her maternal aunts suffered greatly with anxiety. Her father's family had been estranged from one another for years because of angry objections to one sibling's marriage to a woman of mixed race. Alcoholism was rampant. But the detail that completely opened Jackie's eyes was the fact that one grandfather had died as a result of being bipolar. He'd been institutionalized during a manic phase in the winter months, and during the middle of the night had walked out into the cold without clothes on, wandering off for miles before he was found. He died of complications from pneumonia.

That one detail helped to convince Jackie, finally, that her anxiety was not a character flaw or a moral failure; it was in her genes. She realized that what she needed most, in addition to talk therapy, was to bring her brain back into Positive Feedback; that, she hoped, might soothe her nerves and help her release the tension in her neck. And she was right: She quickly found that the Morning Glory ritual, the daily meditation and visualization, the Tibetan Rites, and the shift to anti-inflammatory foods (especially those high in omega-3s) helped calm her anxiety and allowed her to move better and shift more easily into the positive. After a blood test revealed she was extremely low in vitamin D, we found that her calcium level was extremely high. We did an ultrasound and found her parathyroid had started to malfunction. Jackie had started taking high doses of vitamin D, which in turn helped support her parathyroid function and relieve her neck pain. Together we worked on stopping the self-critical thoughts that had been polluting her brain and triggering her sympathetic nervous system, and we substituted powerful positive affirmations that soothed her nerves, shifted her into parasympathetic mode, and helped her deal better with stress.

Soothing her nervous system and strengthening her parasympathetic response is an ongoing process, and Jackie continues to improve month by month. She knows that keeping the commitment to the Morning Glory routine is the best way to signal to her body that all is right with the world. She's hoping that the work she's doing will inspire more of her family members to do their own work, but she's not holding her breath. Either way, she knows that her happiness is *her* responsibility, and she can't help others who don't know how to help themselves.

Some people wonder why I include siblings in the Body Family Tree. I've seen that sometimes their experiences or health scares can serve as a wake-up call for my patients. For example, the sister who has truly awful premenstrual dysphoric disorder may help you understand your mildly awful PMS, while also making you grateful that you don't suffer quite as much; it's all perspective.

BODY TIMELINE

Most of my patients love this exercise. They make big steps forward when they write down their experiences and start to see connections between what happened to them when they were thirteen or eighteen, and now. Those connections are very real and very common.

Often when my patients are suffering from musculoskeletal problems, they're "holding" their pain—their entire musculature has trained itself to guard the injury or the pain, trying to prevent more pain. The problem, of course, is that that pain is then bound up inside the tissues and unable to be released.

I help my patients reflect on their pain—its location and its source—so that they can recognize their own patterns of muscular tension and see how they may be contributing by holding on to the past. Once you recognize the location and origin of your pain, and name it, you're that much closer to releasing it. You really don't need to be clicked and prodded; very subtle changes can have tremendous impact.

The purpose of creating your Body Timeline is multifold: First, you'll recall a lot of information about your own health history that you might have lost or forgotten. Second, it's nice to have all the information in a single place—so you'll never lose it again. And third, my favorite: As you reflect on your body's history, you'll realize just how *much* life you've experienced. The joys, the pains, the sorrows—they're all locked inside your tissues right now, and any pain you might be feeling could be linked directly back to a specific emotional and/or physical experience. And today, any *new* experience—any massage or adjustment or yoga pose, any night of thrilling sex or crushing rejection—might retrigger that memory. How fascinating to do that digging now, and see where today's pains may have begun—and how much life is stored in every single one—so you can appreciate the lessons of each one, process how they've impacted your life, and learn to let them go.

Figure 11. **Example of a Body Timeline**

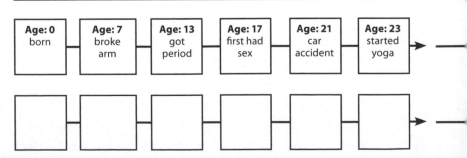

Make a Body Timeline like the one shown in figure 11, but "populate" yours more fully. (The sample, for space reasons, is sparse.) Using separate sheets of paper, make a ten-box timeline for every *decade* of your life (with each box representing a year); note that, unlike the sample, your timeline can contain multiple entries in each box. Start with "Birth" on the first page and end with "Present Day" on the last page. Now start recalling and recording major events in your life:

- Your parents' relationship at your conception

- Your mom's health and stress level during your gestation

- Your birth experience

- The birth of your siblings

- Any known childhood illnesses

- Your early nutrition history

- Your first period

- The first time you had sex

- The first time you were *really* in love

- When you met your partner

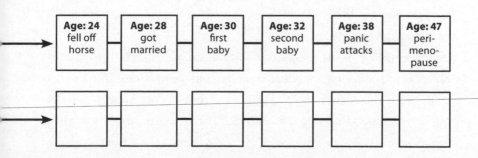

- Your marriage

- Your separation or divorce

- The birth of your first baby

- Your father's death

- A bicycle or skiing accident, or falling off a horse

You get the idea. Place as many emotional and physical experiences as you can recall on the approximate place on your Body Timeline. Don't get too perfectionistic about this. It's not about remembering exactly what year Bobby dumped you for Linda; it's about remembering when the pain in your chest started—the pain that comes back every time you're feeling sad and alone. It's not even about *when* so much as *what*—so you can start to reflect on *what* is still with you, and *why* it is.

You may find that you shed a few tears as you complete this—that is all part of the process. Many people recall deeply painful experiences through this type of exercise. One Ohio State University study found that nearly two-thirds of both men and women reported some type of abuse in their teenage years. More than two-thirds reported two or more abusive partners.[4] These intense experiences can get "forgotten" by your conscious brain in the intervening years; even those that are remembered may be kept to oneself. People often talk themselves out of sharing such experiences even with a counselor or trusted confidante (self-message: "It's really not a big deal"). But even a very "small" trauma—a betrayal by a childhood friend, a taunt on the playground, a cutting remark or appraisal from your parents ("Why can't you be more like your brother?")— can stay with a person for decades. And if *that* level of pain can remain, I'm sure you can believe that the memory of an actual assault could still be locked in your tissues.

This timeline is instrumental in letting the pain speak. Through this exercise, you're finding the source and making connections. Don't be discouraged if the answers aren't readily in front of you. Simply completing the exercise is part of the solution. The reflection itself is healing, and you'll see soon enough the ways in which this timeline will help you better understand your physical and emotional history.

Positive Function

Dr. Still said that structure governs function—and the way we can most impact our function directly is through our diet. But don't dive headlong into some new diet scheme. In this Reflect week, I don't want you to change the foods you're eating. Instead, I want you to spend time reflecting on what you eat and how you eat it. The following exercise will help you with that process.

FOOD DIARY

To gather data, eat as you normally would—every single soda, coffee, cookie, tub of popcorn, everything. Immediately after eating something, write down that food (as in the one-day sample shown in figure 12). You're studying yourself as if you were an animal in the wild: What are her habits? When does she feed?

In your Food Diary, note several things:

- The content of each meal or snack

- The approximate serving size ("breast of chicken" is fine—no need to weigh or measure your food, i.e., not "4 ounces chicken")

- The time of day

- Your emotional mood

- Who was with you (if anyone)

- How you felt afterward, emotionally or physically (do you feel more or less pain?)

Figure 12. **Sample of Food Diary—Before**

DAY	MEAL OR SNACK	CONTENTS OF MEAL	NOTES
Monday	Breakfast	Danish, cappuccino	Delickious, but too sweet—instantly got headache
	Snack	2 more coffees	Zooming by 11 A.M., productive but stressed
	Lunch	Submarine sandwich with ham and cheese	Full and sleepy
	Snack	Coffee, muffin	Snapped at my coworker; amped but can't concentrate
	Dinner	Pasta with meatballs, 3 glasses of wine	Fell asleep on the couch; woke at 3 A.M., hot and anxious

Sample of Food Diary—After

DAY	MEAL OR SNACK	CONTENTS OF MEAL	NOTES
Monday	Breakfast	2 eggs, smoothie	Good energy, but a bit too full
	Snack	Handful of almonds	Ok, a little headache
	Lunch	Romaine lettuce, tomatoes, walnuts, pineapple	Delicious, but could have used a bit more protein
	Snack	2 small apples	Crunchy and sweet— gave me lots of energy
	Dinner	Grilled salmon, steamed spinach with garlic and lemon, tomato salad with green beans	So satisfying—wasn't hungry at night like usual

Try to record your eating for the whole Reflect week, but even three days (the minimum) will give you a wealth of data. It will also help you become more aware of just how much crap—or good stuff!—you're eating. At this stage, most people have a fairly disturbing picture to look at. It can be amazing to realize just how much garbage we typically put into our bodies. You'll also notice if you've been feeding your emotions.

You probably won't want to *record* specific nutrient information, but pay attention to it as you're shopping. The habit of noting such information may actually help you reduce any excess pounds. An international study by researchers from Spain, Norway, Arkansas, and Tennessee, using information from twenty-five thousand observations on health, eating, and shopping habits, found that women who read food labels weigh nearly nine pounds less than women who don't.[5] Whether this difference is the result of reading labels itself or simply a sign of these women's greater orientation toward healthy food, we can't know—but the practice of tracking your food during this week will certainly give you essential data that will help you craft your nutritional approach in the Release and Radiate stages.

MINDFUL EATING

If I can suggest that you do anything different about your nutrition during the Reflect stage, it's that you pay closer attention to eating. The Food Diary is an excellent first step. The second is to eat "mindfully."

Mindful eating is actually a form of meditation. (We'll learn more about meditation in the "Positive Emotion" section below.) When you eat mindfully, you focus with your entire being on the act of eating.

Sound boring? It doesn't have to be—in fact, if you do it right, it can be endlessly fascinating. You'll be actively training your attention on sensory information. By focusing so intently on such a small number of sensory details, you'll help to decrease your distractibility. You'll develop insight, concentration, absorption—all master skills that will help enrich and deepen your experience in other areas of your life.

A few ground rules about mindful eating:

- You must eat at a table, sitting down

- You must not *eat* near a screen of any kind (computer, television, iPhone, or other smart phone or tablet)

- You must put all your food on a plate. If you can manage to use silver cutlery, a nice glass for your water, and a cloth napkin, even better.

- You may eat with other people, but the mindful eating meditation is more easily done on your own (which you'll understand in a second)

- You must give yourself at least thirty minutes to eat your meal

To begin your mindful eating exercise, put your food on your plate, carry it to the table, and sit down. Put your napkin on your lap, and rest your hands on top of it. Close your eyes and take a deep cleansing breath; then say to yourself (or to God or the universe or any higher power):

Thank you for this moment to truly taste and savor my food.

(In case you're reluctant to invoke God or a higher power, let me reassure you that, when meditating, putting yourself into the hands of something or someone "larger than yourself" has therapeutic value in and of itself. Scientists writing in the *Journal of Affective Disorders* found that when those who believe in God undergo therapy, their treatment is more effective. Why? Researchers believe that faith works the same way the placebo effect does: When you believe something will work, it works!)

After your moment of grateful meditation, open your eyes, pick up your fork, and put your first bite into your mouth. Here's where everything really slows down. First, feel the tines of the fork on your lips and tongue; feel how cold the steel or silver is against your tongue. As you place the food in your mouth, notice how your mouth starts to water in expectation of eating it. Bite down slowly, and feel your teeth going through the food and joining with the opposing teeth.

Get the idea? Super slow-mo. Go as slowly as you can, noticing every single sensation, flavor, texture. Name them in your head: Salty. Smooth. Hot. Chewy.

Eat your first few bites like this, and then give yourself a break. Finish the rest of your meal at a slightly faster pace, but still taking care to focus your full attention on your food and to notice as much as you can: How the plate changes as the food disappears. How crumbs appear on the table (how did that happen?). How the flavors seem to morph after a few bites. All the minute details of your meal—notice as many as you can.

This Reflect exercise will have more impact than you can imagine. Research has shown that when overweight people learn and use a mindful eating exercise, they tend to lose weight, feel less stressed and depressed, and have a more optimistic outlook on life, without making any other changes.[6] One study published in the *Journal of the Academy of Nutrition and Dietetics* found that diabetics who did a mindful eating course significantly lowered their A1C (a measure of blood sugar control).[7] Even people with a clinically diagnosed eating disorder tend to show more healthy food habits after learning mindful eating.[8]

When you're busy, mindful eating not only builds in another moment of meditation, it actively trains you to pay attention to *everything* in a more meaningful and more conscious way. You start to sink more deeply into the moment and experience all of the colors and flavors of your life, both at the dinner table and out in the world.

Also, here's a sneaky part: When you lay out the nice china and the cloth napkins, you may find (even though you're not supposed to change the food you're eating this week) that your deli hoagie and Diet Coke don't suit the environment the way they do when you scarf them down in front of the computer. As you continue on with mindful eating, you may notice yourself making selections with slightly more consideration for such aesthetics. But again, that's not the objective during the Reflect stage. For now the objective is simply to notice, to pay attention—to reflect on—the finer points of what you're putting into your body and how it makes you feel.

A Meal Fit For a Queen

So, you say you can't wait: You want to make a change in your food *right now*. Okay, okay—I'll make an exception. But only for breakfast.

Breakfast is my favorite meal of the day and helps me get off on the right foot. Surrounded by the ones I love, I eat a healthy, copious breakfast—one fit for a queen. I feel special, nourishing my body and strengthening my spirit for the day ahead.

My goal in life is to break the addiction many of my patients have to baguettes or white bread toast and coffee for breakfast. What a one-two inflammation punch! When you have white bread with coffee for breakfast, you send your endocrine system reeling: Your cortisol level shoots up alongside your blood sugar level, which prompts a major reaction from your insulin and kicks up your inflammatory response first thing in the morning—not setting the best course for the day.

A breakfast made with eggs, on the other hand, can set you up for a steady release of energy for the morning and into the early afternoon. The protein helps you stay satisfied longer, so you can concentrate better and resist temptation throughout the day.

With a belly full of energy-enhancing, nutritious food—any of the meals fit for a queen below—you can begin to do the hard work necessary to really dig into the whole picture. Bonus: Many of these anti-inflammatory foods will be incorporated into the Release stage, just in smaller quantities. Trying them now, in larger portion sizes, introduces your taste buds to their loveliness but doesn't leave you with a sense of deprivation. All your energy should be focused on reflection this week—there will be time enough for release later.

Here are some ideas for your five-star Reflection breakfast. Try all five this week:

Smoothie: Mix goat's-milk yogurt with a handful of blueberries, raspberries, and some pineapple chunks; add 1 tablespoon coconut oil along with a few almonds or a handful of walnuts and some ice (if desired). Blend the mixture until you achieve the consistency you like.

Oatmeal: Cook some steel-cut whole-grain oats with walnuts, cinnamon, 1 tablespoon coconut oil, and 1 cup almond milk; sprinkle ½ tablespoon cocoa powder and 1 tablespoon each goji berries, organic milled flaxseed, chia seeds, and sweet manuka honey (which has antibacterial properties).

Eggs: Make a three-egg (whites only) omelet with goat's-milk feta cheese, thyme, and tomatoes. (Goat's milk has less lactose than cow's milk, as well as different proteins, and thus is less inflammatory.)

Bread: Top two slices Ezekiel bread (wheat-free and if possible yeast-free) with pure almond butter and sliced banana. Sprinkle on some goji berries.

Beverage: Enjoy one coffee after breakfast with almond milk and a sprinkle of cinnamon. For the rest of the day, green tea or nettle tea will give you energy, purify your system, and move excess fluids toward elimination.

Positive Motion

We've talked about how the Reflect component of the Positive Feedback program is really about taking stock, not making changes. The one change you'll be making to your day-to-day schedule, as noted earlier in this chapter, is the addition of the Morning Glory ritual, including the Tibetan Rites of Rejuvenation exercises. If you've already been quite active, the Tibetan Rites should be no problem for you. But if you've been basically sedentary for a while, know that even this small amount of exercise could do tremendous benefit. Doctors from the Mayo Clinic claim that even as little as ten minutes a day of exercise can reduce your risk of heart disease by 50 percent.[9] As we move into weeks 2 and 3 of the program, you will add other exercise routines and challenges that help to further tone your Adaptive Response. Getting into the rhythm of the daily Morning Glory routine now, during the Reflect stage, will set you up for that expanded exercise routine.

Positive Emotion

Honest emotion is the root of all health. When we have positive emotion, we are better able to do the work that gives us positive structure, function, and motion. Being honest about our emotion, particularly that which is negative, is the core work of the Reflect stage. And among the self-care categories we're discussing here—structure, function, motion, and emotion—emotion is typically where most of the work *needs* to be done. We hold ourselves back because of painful emotions that we're not facing, let alone expressing.

Once you find the courage to reveal those buried emotions to yourself and the world, you can tackle any physical challenge that comes along. The work it takes to move yourself back into the positive will become a joyful challenge and exploration, as opposed to an insurmountable burden.

POSITIVE SELF-TALK

One of the most common ways that people keep themselves in the negative is with their internal dialogue. You may not realize that you have a constant din of negative patter going on inside your head, but chances are you do. Perhaps you believe that things are all black or all white, all good or all bad—and, just your luck, you've gotten all the bad stuff. Why? Chances are you'll zero in on yourself to answer that question, assuming that you "caused" your situation to go bad.

Far too many of us live in a jail of our own creation. Most often, when we're in Negative Feedback, we're not talking to ourselves with love; we're talking to ourselves in a harsh, judgmental way. Chronic negative self-talk triggers an amygdala response and activates the SNS needlessly. And we keep that pattern going every time we have a negative thought. Why do we do this to ourselves? If there's one place in the world where you should get the benefit of the doubt, it's in your own mind!

This internal patter is yet another sign of unresolved injury or pain that lives within the brain. At some point, you may have heard and internalized a negative judgment about yourself. Perhaps your mother constantly commented unkindly on your appearance. Maybe your dad called you lazy or teased you in a sarcastic way that stuck. Or maybe a teacher said you weren't "living up to your potential." Sometimes comments like this can roll off our backs; other times, the smallest comment can stick with us and make us cringe and squirm years later. The person who made the comment may not have any memory of the words spoken, but their damage was done (and remains). The worst part of this is when you stop hearing those words in *another* person's voice and they simply become the background noise of your life: *You're fat/lazy/ stupid/boring.* And if you've listened to those comments for years and years, you might not even recognize them anymore—they've simply become your truth.

Try this: Close your eyes and imagine that you're getting dressed to go out for a big night. You look in your closet for something to wear.

What are you saying to yourself at that moment? Does it sound something like this?

> You're too fat for that dress, too old for those boots. All your clothes are outdated. You're going to look like a fool whatever you wear. Why even bother? What makes you think you have anything interesting to say to those people anyway?

Or does it sound something like this?

> Wow, you look amazing: Your energy is sparkling right through. The color of that sweater is beautiful on you. The people who sit next to you tonight are going to be amazed by your brilliance. You're going to be the belle of the ball! Bet you can't wait to get there!

Did you giggle a little at this last paragraph? Perhaps it seems conceited to think of yourself in those terms? But compare those two paragraphs: They're roughly equivalent in intensity of tone, though at opposite ends of the spectrum. Why is it so hard to think of yourself in glowing terms, whereas a correspondingly negative attitude seems perfectly normal (if a bit depressing)?

If your thoughts resemble the first paragraph more closely than the last, you must *learn* to stop such thoughts and immediately replace trash talk with positive words. Take a moment to reflect on your internal self-talk and write down in your notebook what you're saying to yourself. (The mindfulness skills that you worked on during your mindful eating exercise can help you here.) Finish these sentences:

> My body is . . .
>
> My mind is . . .
>
> The things I love about me are . . .
>
> The things I want to change about me are . . .

Write them quickly, without censoring yourself.

Once they're on the page, look at them critically. By noticing these thoughts and trying to capture them while you disengage from the emotional content, you can start to realize how harsh you're being with yourself.

You don't have to go all Pollyanna or "I'm great" if it's uncomfortable— though this thought-swapping likely *will* feel awkward at first—but confronting your interior monologue is the only way to seize control of your unconscious negative thoughts and replace them with powerful attitudes that will give you strength. Consider these thought-pairings:

You're too fat for that outfit.	⮕	I like this and it feels comfortable; this is my uniform. I feel safe, which is what is important.
All your clothes are outdated.	⮕	Thank goodness I don't have to buy trendy clothes to feel good about myself.
You're going to look like a fool.	⮕	No one is going to be worried about looking at me; they're all going to be worried about themselves.
Why even bother?	⮕	I deserve this night out. I deserve to feel good in my skin, and to feel beautiful.

Simply by reflecting on your negative thoughts—even if you can't bring yourself to counter them just yet—you'll begin to see and understand that you *don't* have to believe your negative assessments; you *can* make an entirely new choice. You are in control; you have the power to change the way you *feel* by changing the words you *think*.

This might feel awkward and heavy-handed at first, but thought-switching has been repeatedly proven to reduce anxiety and obsessive thinking, and to improve self-confidence.[10] In fact, with repeated use of

Table 5. **Time Audit Template**

HOUR	ACTIVITY	EMOTION
6:00 A.M.		
7:00 A.M.		
8:00 A.M.		
9:00 A.M.		
10:00 A.M.		
11:00 A.M.		
12:00 P.M.		
1:00 P.M.		
2:00 P.M.		
3:00 P.M.		
4:00 P.M.		
5:00 P.M.		
6:00 P.M.		
7:00 P.M.		
8:00 P.M.		
9:00 P.M.		
10:00 P.M.		

Figure 13. **Sample of Time Audit**

HOUR	ACTIVITY	EMOTION
6:00 A.M.	Wake, shower	Sleepy, optimistic
7:00 A.M.	Get kids ready for day care	Rushed, playful
8:00 A.M.	Commute to work	Bored, annoyed, angry
9:00 A.M.	First meeting	Excited, anxious
10:00 A.M.	Coffee break	Happy, laughing
11:00 A.M.	Project work	Focused, frustrated
12:00 P.M.	Lunch	Rushed, self-conscious
1:00 P.M.	Conference call	Bored, frustrated, confused
2:00 P.M.	E-mail	Stressed, amused
3:00 P.M.	Project work	Distracted, "brain fog"
4:00 P.M.	Project work	Focused, "in the zone"
5:00 P.M.	Leave for day care	Relieved, tired, excited
6:00 P.M.	Cooking dinner	Distracted, irritable
7:00 P.M.	Eating dinner	Happy, relaxed, loved
8:00 P.M.	Bath/bedtime	Relaxed, tired, impatient
9:00 P.M.	Facebook, Netflix	Zoned out, weary, slightly depressed
10:00 P.M.	Lights out	Bone-tired, yet anxious and keyed-up

this exercise, you'll change the actual neurochemistry and structure of your brain to favor more positive thoughts; simply put, you'll train your brain to be happier and more confident.[11]

TIME AUDIT

Time is the essence of our lives. Time is the one resource we can never get back once it's gone. But many of us squander much of our lives doing things that we don't really *want* to do—we just do them out of habit. To see how *you* do in using your time, take a Time Audit, an exercise that tracks your activities. (See the sample in figure 13.)

When you've completed your Time Audit, you may be shocked at how much time you spend online, watching television, stalking ex-boyfriends on Facebook, or checking-checking-checking e-mail and Twitter—things you don't even know you're doing or really want to do. Be warned: You might get partway through this exercise and be tempted to stop because the results are so surprising (and not in a good way). Many folks realize with a shock that they've been simply sleepwalking through their lives, spending next to zero time on projects or people that really matter to them. But, as painful as it might be, calling attention to how you've been squandering your time can help bring you back into the present. This dawning realization of the quantity of time wasted is one of the core reasons people unconsciously opt to live in pain: The awareness of the loss of that time can be so devastating that they prefer not to address or accept it.

Again, as with your Food Diary, don't drastically alter anything about your day-to-day existence while you complete your Time Audit. (Although, inevitably, the mere act of writing down what you do makes you spend your time more wisely—a lesson in itself!) But the objective here is to collect data. You want to see what you're doing with your time when you're not focused on just how precious it is.

Make three copies of the blank chart shown in table 5 (or print them out at elixirliving.com), one for each of three days of data collection, and paste them in your program notebook or put them in your three-ring binder. Keep them with you at all times so that you can track your activities.

AFFIRMATIONS AND MEDITATIONS

You may already have guessed that you're going to do a lot of affirmations and meditations on the Positive Feedback plan. Often my new patients roll their eyes and give me a "Do I have to?" whine about these, as if they were just a silly waste of time. But believe me, *these are not optional.* They *work.* They help you reprogram your brain, one affirmation and prayer and meditation at a time. My most successful patients, the Grammy-Oscar-Tony winners, the heads of state and multinational corporations, the amazingly creative and talented artists—they all meditate at least once, twice, or even three times a day. These busy folks force themselves to find those few minutes because those brief pauses pay back such enormous benefits in clarity, focus, productivity, and peace.

Meditation is a miracle that makes it possible for you to control your body and your health with your mind. The research is overwhelming: Meditation decreases stress hormones, insomnia, recurrence of depression, anxiety and panic, blood pressure, and many other debilitating diseases and conditions.[12] At the same time, it also increases focus, concentration, memory, contentment, immunity, blood sugar control—even the very *size* of your brain—and more.[13] When meditation is sustained long enough, it can turn back the clock on your genes, preserving the length of telomeres, the caps at the end of your chromosomes that protect them from fraying, and in so doing, guard against aging and disease.[14] One study found that just twelve minutes a day of meditation for eight weeks increased anti-aging telomerase activity by 46 percent.[15] Researchers are not entirely sure how meditation is responsible for all these physical benefits, but they suspect it has something to do with reducing activity in the sympathetic nervous system and increasing activity in the parasympathetic nervous system.[16] All these benefits from sitting quietly for fewer than fifteen minutes a day. Amazing!

Perhaps the biggest effect I've seen is what meditation can do to relieve pain. Meditation is about finding your own power and believing in yourself. Many women are able to deliver their children by tapping into this amazing innate power. One Wake Forest University study found that meditation can have a stronger effect on pain than *morphine!* Most pain-relieving drugs reduce pain by about 25 percent. This study found that meditation reduced pain intensity by 40 percent and pain unpleasantness by 57 percent after just one hour of meditation training.[17] The subjects did a form of mindfulness meditation: Whatever sensation or thought came to them while meditating, they would consider it, label it ("worry," "hunger"), and then release it. The study researchers learned that the meditation caused multiple reactions throughout the brain. For example, they found (via brain scans) that it triggered the orbitofrontal cortex, a part of the brain involved in reframing pain perceptions, and thus reduced the unpleasantness of pain. Meditation also quieted the activity of the hypothalamus, basically heading off any messages to the amygdala and putting a cool-off period between the sensory input and executive brain function.

Meditation is like a highly potent antistress serum—it increases the activity of the laid-back parasympathetic nervous system while it simultaneously cools down the hot-headed sympathetic nervous system. As a result, your entire body—not just your emotions—can calm down after stress more quickly and efficiently, cooling off your inflammation and reducing the wear and tear on your tissues. Thus meditation is a very effective tool for you in the Positive Feedback program, and one that you should use all day long. I want you to come away from this book knowing that meditation can change your brain and alter how your body reacts to stress. It's a greater, more powerful instrument of health than almost any medicine on earth.

While some purist meditators might find this sacrilegious, I like to pair the calm, open space of meditation with powerful affirmations—positive statements constructed in a way that can break through mental blocks and change long-standing negative thought patterns. I find that our brains are at their most receptive at moments of quiet, meditative stillness. For that reason, "installing" powerful affirmative ways of thinking is much more effective when we're at peace and our negative thoughts have been cleared away.

As I mentioned earlier, you can adopt any of the meditations and affirmations included in this book. In addition, though, you'll want to create your own, targeting your personal needs and goals. The more personally meaningful to you, the more positive and potent the effects.

Meditation is really just a simple breathing exercise. You can sit in any quiet space—in the bathtub, in your car, in your office—close your eyes, breathe deeply in and out of your nose, and say something like the following to yourself:

This is *me* time. I am reconnecting with my cells, relaxing my
muscles, and helping my nerves feel less tension. I am reflecting
on where I am; I am helping my brain calm down from worry.
I am talking to myself, my brain: I am safe. I am strong. I am
calm. I am at peace.

When you're creating a meditation or positive affirmation, the key is
to get right to the heart of what's holding you back. Let's consider an
example:

Cristina was having trouble growing beyond her preconceived notions
of her own ability. Through her work with her Body Timeline, she realized
that she was stuck in fear and unable to grow because of a deeply ingrained
faulty self-image. She had been raised to be a wife, but not to have her own
life, her own passion. Now she was lost in her own unfulfilled dreams. This
meditation is an example of the kind that helped her find her confidence:

I grow beyond where I am today. I exceed beyond my parents
and teachers. I live for myself. I dream. I visualize. I ask for the
right man or husband. I release the past. I believe in myself, and
my dreams come true.

I truly believe that if you don't believe in yourself with passion and
discipline, nobody can help you. That's why building yourself up with
the Morning Glory ritual and crafting very specific meditations is so important. If you really believe in yourself, what you wish for *will come true
for you.* Even if it's a tough journey, you have to stay in the positive and
things will unfold for the best.

Morning meditation.
When I meditate in the morning, as part of the Morning Glory routine,
it's about clearing my mind and starting my day positively:

Okay, this is a good start to the day. I feel positive. This day is a
new beginning. I attract the positive; good things can and will
happen to me.

Sometimes—and it happens to all us—we start the day with negative thoughts. Whether it's some*thing* or some*one,* we're worried and upset before we even get out of bed. Instead of allowing a cloud to hang over our head, we can turn to a positive meditation:

> Okay, I have something negative in my mind. I am feeling [state concern]. I have control over this feeling, and I can free myself. This negativity does not have the power to ruin my day. I am in control, and I will work on it. Things are going to be okay. I am focusing on all the positives and finding the calm to attract positive things.

My morning meditation sets the tone for my day and helps me prepare for any negative things I can anticipate. It's like a morning vaccine: I'm building up positive antibodies to fend off the day's incoming negative viruses.

Afternoon meditation.

My afternoon meditation is done during stolen time. I try to find ten to fifteen minutes of quiet *me* time in between patients and running to pick up my boys from school. I see it as a simple breathing exercise, and I think to myself:

> I close my eyes; I reconnect with my cells. I relax my muscles and help my nerves feel less tension. I reflect on where I am, helping my brain calm down from worry and tension. I talk directly to my brain. I am safe; I am strong; I am not sick. I grow beyond and I exceed my parents and my teachers. I live for myself. I release the past. I believe in myself and my dreams are coming true.

My afternoon meditation is more of a visualization of what I'd like to have happen:

> I am strong. I close my eyes and connect with my power. I am clear and my brain is creative: I finish my project and feel

confident and happy with the result. I am productive and happy and proud of my work.

Evening meditation.

The evening meditation/affirmation is all about reflecting on the day. What went well? What am I grateful for? What would I have preferred not to have happened? Evening meditation is about getting rid of all the bad and recognizing the good:

> My husband and I had a squabble today, but we are done
> with that. I forgive him and he forgives me. We are rid of
> that argument. Please help me release from pain—physical,
> emotional, conscious, unconscious. I forgive all the people who
> have hurt me.

Evening meditation is also about loosening your grip and realizing you don't have control over other people:

> Please let me or help me forgive people who have hurt me.
> I want to send them love so that we can both be free. I release
> the need to control [partner's name]. I celebrate his uniqueness
> and our love and respect for each other. I do not try to
> change him.

In reflective meditation, it's important that you acknowledge your grudges, your anger, and your pain.

> I ask for forgiveness from myself, from all people, all ego, all
> anger, all children, for all the universe and its ancestors. All
> people forgive each other. God [or the universe or nothing], I
> am full of gratitude. God, give me all the love, peace, and joy.
> Thank you, God. Thank you, body.

At the end of each day, remember to use your positive sleep strategy and commit to those seven to eight hours of quality sleep every night. Restorative sleep will help build up your system so that you're less emotionally reactive and more able to calmly assess your feelings and not carry them around with you. The less reactive you are to immediate annoyances, the more energy you have to delve deeply into your issues during week 1 and get ready for the intense work of week 2.

Check-In: Are You Ready to Release?

Now that you're at the end of your Reflect week, you're probably chomping at the bit to jump into the Release stage. Having spent the better part of this week really facing your pain, you may be incredibly motivated to make huge changes. If that sounds like you, fantastic. But before you leap ahead, I want to check in and make sure that you've completed some of the critical pieces of the Reflect stage, because they give you the raw material to work with in the Release and Radiate stages.

Have you committed to getting seven to eight hours of sleep every night, and have you woken up with the Morning Glory ritual at least three days this week? Do you feel like those habits are becoming fairly solid and a part of your everyday routine?

Have you completed your Body Map, Body Family Tree, and Body Timeline? Have you begun to notice some patterns and connections there?

Have you practiced mindful eating at least twice (or even three times)? Did you have an "ah-hah!" moment when you savored your food fully for the first time in months?

Have you filled out the Food Diary and Time Audit for at least three days? Were you honest with yourself? Did you include all the junk food and time-wasters that might embarrass you? (If not, please do the work again before moving on. Facing the pain of reality, especially when it comes to wasted time, is a critical part of your breakdown-to-breakthrough transition.)

If you've answered yes to most of these questions, I'm thrilled. That means you're ready to let all your pain and negativity go. Let's turn to the Release stage and put your newfound information and resolve to work.

Week 2: Release

Anything I cannot transform into
something marvelous, I let go.

—Anaïs Nin

Most people come to my office looking for release. Put another way, release is the primary purpose for most of the visits in my practice. People want to get rid of the bad junk in their bodies and their lives.

Most often, they want to lie down on my table and get up again half an hour later refreshed and renewed. They want *my work* to enable them to skip out of my office, leaving behind all their negative energy. I do my best to help them feel better right away, because I know that pain can blind a person to forward progress. But the most successful patients know that the true work is really *up to them*. I can provide momentary release with a treatment, but that effect will last only one or two days.

As is the case with those patients, only *you* can do the work to create a full release that will change your life. By following the Release protocol outlined in this chapter, you'll systematically begin to let go of all that doesn't serve you: the inflammation-causing foods in your diet, the toxins in your muscles and skin, the waste buildup in your lymphatic and glymphatic systems, the habits that get in the way of your life, and the pain that's been hampering your every move. In addition, and this is vital, you will get rid of the negative energy that's pulling you and your choices in a downward spiral. By releasing the negative in this chapter, you will regain your power and step back into your body—as my patient Kerry did.

Kerry was one of the most beautiful women I'd ever seen. At forty-five, she had endearing smile lines around her big brown eyes. When she did smile, her entire face lit up from her brilliant white teeth.

When she came in to see me, though, she wasn't smiling. She had been contending with fatigue and general aches and pains, and she was hoping for some kind of cure. A disciplined woman, she went to the gym every day and did yoga and stretching religiously. But her pains remained, and she said they were starting to interfere with her marriage. She said she and her husband hadn't made love in months. I sent her home with my program and asked her to come back the following week.

As we went over her Body Timeline, a few things jumped out at me. For one thing, she'd been very trim and "healthy" her whole life—she'd never smoked and had maintained a steady body weight since high school (partially by drinking four cans of diet soda a day). She worked hard to take care of herself. But since marrying her husband, she'd had several accidents: She fell off her bike. She broke a toe. She sprained a wrist. What was happening?

When we looked at her Time Audit, I was astonished at how much time she spent exercising and taking care of her home. She rose at four forty-five every morning to go to the gym for two hours, then returned home to get the kids ready for school, worked a full day in her home office, oversaw homework, and then did three or four hours of house-work. Sometimes she wouldn't get to bed until after midnight—a tough bedtime for someone who gets up well before dawn!

I could see the toll this lifestyle was taking on her. In addition to the chronic pain, her blood tests showed that she was trending toward anemia. Her hair was getting thin, and under her expertly applied makeup, I could see dark circles under her eyes.

I asked her to redo her Time Audit, but this time to use the Release the Time-Wasters exercise (which we'll look at later in this chapter) as part of her Release work. Together we worked on revising her audit. With the schedule changed on paper, the housework and gym time were greatly reduced. Kerry reluctantly promised to honor those revisions and spend more time with her daughters and girlfriends and outside among nature. She would hike more and fold laundry less.

Okay, I said, now it's time to make this ideal Time Audit happen. But I could tell, from her reluctance to commit, that something more was happening with those late-night chores. I decided to dig in as to why she was working so hard. I asked her if she could let some of that stuff slip a bit. She shook her head.

"He'd never let me," she said, looking down.

Hmmm. "How about the gym—could you skip that a few days a week, and just take a walk? You could use some more sleep."

"That's our deal," she said, shaking her head. A tear slipped out of one huge brown eye, and then many more followed. I waited until her tears stopped and she started talking.

What the Time Audit allowed Kerry to release was something she'd been holding deep inside for far too long: She confessed that her husband was very controlling, trying to dictate every step of her life, including the insistence that she maintain a perfect size-2 body at all costs. He had paid for her to redo her teeth, routinely selected her hairstyle and color, chose her clothes, and even insisted that she get a facelift at forty-two. This same unreasonable standard of perfection was imposed upon their home, which demanded dozens of hours of labor a week to maintain to his satisfaction. Kerry confessed that they hadn't had sex in a year, but she was starting to be attracted to men at the gym.

Every week Kerry came in to see me for a treatment, but more important, she was sticking to the program and getting physically and emotionally stronger. I saw a gradual loosening of her shoulders, a fading of those black circles, a brightening of her eyes. As she released her addiction to diet soda, got more sleep, and stopped working her body so hard, the inflammation that had kept her joints in pain started to recede. Her movements became more fluid, her smile easier and more genuine. Before too long, she declared that she wanted out of her marriage.

Six months later, she was a free woman. She and her ex had worked out a custody-sharing agreement, and she suddenly had three or four days a week all to herself—heavenly space to explore all her long-neglected interests. Kerry found a beautiful house that she wanted to refurbish—but in her own time. She confessed to me with a giggle that she left piles of laundry around the house now—just because she could. She wasn't quite sure what the next chapter of her life would hold—she was starting to explore that in her Radiate work—but for now, she was quite happy to be released, in every sense of the word.

Letting It Go

When patients come into my office, I can use any number of treatments to help them release the pain quickly. With acupuncture needles, I can either work on the nerves locally, to release trigger points, or remotely, by placing the needles close to specific segments of the spinal cord where the nerves reach into the central nervous system. Whichever method I use, these needles trigger multiple effects within the body, one of which is to release beneficial hormones (such as feel-good endorphins and the cuddle hormone, oxytocin) into the cerebral spinal fluid and blood supply. These natural chemicals help reduce inflammation, lower blood pressure, stimulate positive brain waves, relax the nerves, and more.

All of these effects are also available to you in your own home. The reaction to dry brushing or meditation or trigger-point self-massage may not be as immediately dramatic as an acupuncture treatment, but these self-care options are available to you at any time—*you* are in control of where and when and how often you use them. You don't have to find a practitioner or spend hundreds of dollars; you can experience release using materials found in your own home. And when you combine several of these self-care choices into your full Positive Feedback program, the results will last *much* longer. These biochemical changes compound one another, rebuilding your body's Adaptive Response and bringing you back into the positive.

Perhaps the most important element of the Release stage is to *believe* you have this power to heal yourself. You don't need to be an osteopath to make release happen. To be honest, when I'm preparing for a session, I don't think about the science: I think about releasing energy.

Here's my pretreatment ritual: I say a prayer before the session. I light a candle, which my patients can see when they enter the treatment room. But I also place a glass of water underneath the treatment table, which they *can't* see—that's just for me. I believe that the water can absorb some of the negative energy flowing out of their body. I use my intuition to guide me in releasing their pain. Some of it passes through me as well: During the session, as I feel the energy flowing through their tissues and into my hands, I often find myself yawning or burping! It's as if the pain and bad energy had transformed into gas, and my body was releasing it, getting it out in any way possible.

Now . . . does that sound a little "out there"? Possibly a little crazy? Perhaps. But here's the thing: These methods of release work for me and, more important, for my patients. Whether the methods are scientifically verifiable is absolutely immaterial. Because I believe that the energy is being released, my brain tells my body it can be calm and stay loose. I can be present with my patients and help them release their pain without feeling like I have to keep up my boundaries and barriers. This relaxed openness makes me a better healer, and it also makes me a stronger person.

In my heart, I have faith that these rituals tap into an all-powerful protective spirit, and that spirit prevents me from getting drawn into bad energy. But, devil's advocate: Let's just say I'm wrong and somewhere out in the universe is proof that there is *no* all-powerful protective spirit. That wouldn't make any difference in how powerful these methods are for me! Call it the placebo effect (as noted earlier), call it divine intervention, call it fate—using the candle and the water as protection for my soul works for me simply *because* I believe in it.

This tranquil faith works in tandem with scientifically verifiable approaches to help me release my patients. This combination of science and belief also keeps my body in a positive state, letting me stay strong enough to protect myself from harmful influences of all kinds. This approach is my personal recipe for positive release. Because I've experienced it so many times to great effect, my faith grows ever stronger—which makes the effects even stronger. Behold, the Positive Feedback loop in action!

You don't need to believe in a higher power for the Positive Feedback plan to work. All you need is faith in your own power to heal yourself. If you're ready to move into the positive, I have a very simple program to do the elemental work to cleanse and release the toxins from your structure, function, motion, and emotion. Let's look at each of these areas, one at a time, and discuss strategies you can use to release the negativity in each.

Positive Structure

We've talked a lot about the traumas that remain locked in your tissues for years if they're not released. These don't have to be *major* traumas, either—they can be the childhood memory of an insult muttered under a mean girl's breath, a constant low-grade worry about losing your job, or simply the chronic stress of your everyday life. Repeated triggering of your sympathetic nervous system and the resulting cascade of stress hormones leave an indelible trace of inflammation in your body. NIH researchers found that these stresses can change us down to a genetic level! Researchers studied fifty women, half of them caring for people with Alzheimer's disease, and found that the telomeres of the most stressed women were shorter, leaving the genes more exposed to damage. In effect, their genes were older than their actual age. The genes of the women who reacted most dramatically to minor stresses—such as making a speech or figuring out a tough math problem—seemed older than the genes of those who had a more muted stress response. The caregivers' stress response was most pronounced. The researchers concluded that it was their chronic, unrelenting responsibility that primed their stress response and made them more reactive.[1] When your SNS is triggered by worry and overwork too often, you more easily move from alert to alarm at any moment. Those who don't react so strongly spend more time in a composed, relaxed state—and have "younger," more protected genes as a result.

Despite our culture's emphasis on productivity, deep rest and the ability to relax shouldn't be seen as simply a welcome escape or an indulgence. Indeed, the ability to relax is essential for baseline health. Without that time to release our responsibilities and our troubles, our nervous system never has a chance to reset to normal levels and we stay in the red zone, ready to "blow" at any moment.

Trying to shift this habit from keyed up to calmed down is the core of the Positive Feedback plan. Negative thoughts trigger the stress response just as much as negative situations do. That stress response creates muscle tension in your face and body, which in turn creates more negative thinking. But actively relaxing your facial and body muscles coaxes your brain in the opposite direction. Not only does your body feel more relaxed, but your heart rate slows down and your levels of cortisol and other stress hormones start to even out. In particular, the slowing of your breath helps your entire body to relax and calm down. If you can do only one thing to help yourself release, focus on your breathing—slowing it down, paying attention to the way each breath comes in and goes out of your body, allowing yourself to "hit the bottom" of your lungs, all to trigger your parasympathetic reflex. In this way, you take what's normally an automatic biological response and turn it into walking meditation.

But you're *not* restricted to just one Release technique. Let's look at a few other means of helping your body release pent-up muscular tension and trauma in the structure of your body.

SELF-HEALING TRIGGER POINTS

While I would like nothing more than to be able to give a hands-on treatment to you one-on-one, I'll instead share a self-help method that *you* can use to tap into your body's internal healing mechanisms and Release your pain *with your own hands:* self-healing trigger points, shown in the front and back illustrations of figure 14. These are the same trigger points that

I use in my massage, acupuncture, and cranial sacral treatments with patients. Using a very specific technique (described below) at these trigger points, you'll be able to press the PAUSE button on Negative Feedback, momentarily break the cycle of your pain, and allow yourself the space and the rest to step back and look at what your pain is trying to tell you.

At these trigger points, your fingers can take the place of, say, an acupuncture needle. Points A through N on the front of the body are the easiest to access by yourself. Back-body points A through O are best accessed by another person. Ask a friend to swap treatments with you. If you can't find a willing taker, go ahead and try to reach those points yourself—but don't contort yourself to the point that you undermine your own relaxation. Table 6 describes which trigger point have which effects and, in some cases, offers supplemental instructions.

Important: Trigger-point release is *not* massage; thus your hands should not be spread out. Instead, release the trigger point with your thumb. (This also works with localized tender spots that are more irritable than normal.). To release correctly, apply gentle pressure with your thumb, holding it flat, and moving it slowly in a circular motion. Unless otherwise stated in the chart, continue that motion for five seconds and release. Repeat until you feel that the resistance is gone (that is, when you notice that the muscle isn't as tight and your thumb can go deeper, generally about five times); then gently move toward another area of muscle tightness or resistance close by.

Try to incorporate trigger-point release into your day when you first wake up, before you go to sleep, and anytime during the day that you need release. These points not only help you give yourself immediate pain relief, they also help you make the connection that *you* are the most powerful healing force in your life; *you* are your own best doctor, your own most intuitive osteopath. All the healing power you could ever need is right in your own body. These trigger points help you access that power quickly and effectively so that you can focus your attention and efforts on reflecting on and releasing the true source of your pain. (To identify which self-healing trigger points are best to release specific pains and illnesses, check out chapter 9, "The Positive Feedback Remedies.")

Figure 14. **Self-Healing Trigger Points**

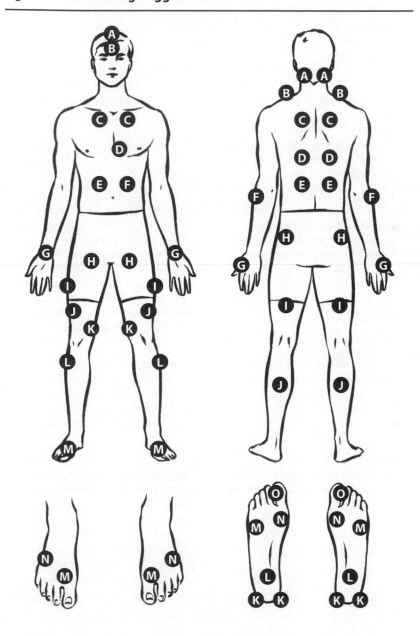

Table 6. **Working with Self-Healing Trigger Points**

TRIGGER POINTS	NOTES
A **Front-Body** Count eight fingers upward from Front B. Apply gentle pressure with your index finger until you find the tender trigger point. Apply steady pressure to that spot, pressing for ten seconds. Take a deep breath in and close your eyes; feel the release as the pain slowly goes away.	This point helps headaches if combined with Back G. Front A also helps with releasing any anger and tension.
Back-Body Count four to five fingers from the back of the ear to Back A, aiming toward the hairline at base of skull. Use the left hand for the left side (and vice versa). Apply gentle pressure with your left thumb and index finger. You will feel a dip and a tender point.	This point helps blood supply to the brain, face, and middle ear and relieves tension headaches, sinus issues, insomnia, tiredness, dizziness, fear, and confusion. (If you have someone doing trigger-point work on you, for this point you can either sit up or lie face-down on your front with your forearms under your forehead.)
B **Front-Body** Sometimes called the "third eye," this is the point between your eyebrows. Apply gentle pressure here.	This point clears the mind and fosters calm and relaxation. It's good for premenstrual anger, combined with Back G and Front M. For panic attacks, combine it with Front C and D, and then with Back G and Front M.
Back-Body This point is halfway between the tip of your shoulder and your neck crease.	This is a gallbladder point. Chinese medicine states that this point helps control judgment and courage. It helps with local muscle pain coming from carrying heavy bags, emotional insecurity, fear of loss of power or control, and generally carrying the world on your shoulders. Helps to let go of overload.

Table 6. **Working with Self-Healing Trigger Points** (continued)

TRIGGER POINTS	NOTES
C **Front-Body** This point is under the clavicle and above your first rib. Count two fingers down from the hollow spot and then two fingers to either side. You will feel a slight dip. Try to hold pressure there for ten seconds. If it feels bruised, that's a good sign, meaning you're on the trigger point. Hold until the feeling of the "bruise" starts to disappear. (But be sure you don't *cause* a bruise from the pressure.)	This point helps with shortness of breath, opens up the throat area, and addresses premenstrual and perimenopausal symptoms, panic attacks, anxiety, grief, sadness, and inability to verbally articulate your thoughts (helps you "spit them out"). This point calms the mind and relieves inflammation.
Back-Body This point is below shoulder level. From the top of the shoulder, count down four fingers, ending up at a level between the fourth and fifth vertebrae.	This point helps release inner chaos or bitterness and helps you forgive and feel free. It also helps with any panic, sadness, and shock after an accident.
D **Front-Body** Place the top of your palm just between the two Front C points and count eight fingers down to Front D, your so-called heart point.	This point is good for anxiety, panic, and shortness of breath that comes with a shock. It helps you focus. It can also help if you're premenstrual and you feel sadness, shortness of breath, or fear.
Back-Body Pretend you place a ruler across your back at the base of your shoulder blades. This point is on this line, on either side of the spine.	This point opens up the diaphragm and helps with pain relief coming from anger or heartbreak. It also helps with negative emotions and fear of the future (anxiety, panic attacks, etc.). Point D is your "diaphragm release point"—it helps you stop holding your breath and aids lymphatic drainage.

Table 6. **Working with Self-Healing Trigger Points** *(continued)*

TRIGGER POINTS	NOTES
E Front-Body Place both your hands around the thinnest part of your waist close to your ribcage (your "solar plexus"). The Front E is on your right.	This point helps with anger release, premenstrual tension, and shortness of breath (diaphragm release).
Back-Body Holding your hands at your waist, as described above, the two Back E points are at your thumbs, but one to two fingers up.	This point helps relieve tiredness, nourish blood, strengthen the heart, and relieve insomnia, lower back pain, and hip pain. Combine it with Back H, I, and J for best lower back pain relief. If you have stomach bloatedness, combine Back E with Front E and F and then follow it down to Front L to clear the stomach channel.
F Front-Body Apply gentle pressure on the left-front lower ribcage area. Try to imagine a straight line down from your left nipple to your lower rib cage. As your index finger finds the tender trigger point, slowly hold pressure for ten seconds. Take a deep breath; as you breathe out, you will feel the release.	This point helps with stomach bloating, loss of appetite, insomnia, and shortness of breath, as well as lymphatic drainage.
Back-Body Find this point while sitting on a chair or on the floor, or lying on your back. Bend your arm or rest it on your desk at a ninety-degree angle. Use your left thumb for the right elbow (and vice versa). Follow the line or crease of the elbow. Start to apply pressure with your thumb two fingers from bony area F, working your way down the middle of the arm toward your index finger, aiming close to Back G. Move slowly down the forearm. Press for ten seconds at each spot until you feel a release and the bruise-like feeling goes away. Keep breathing in and out through your nose; breathe the pain out.	This point helps with constipation, relaxes the large intestine, and relieves bloatedness. A so-called energy point, it also helps with lymphatic drainage.

Table 6. **Working with Self-Healing Trigger Points** (continued)

TRIGGER POINTS	NOTES
G Front-Body Apply your right three fingers flat to the crease of your left wrist (and vice versa). Use your thumb to find the midline close to your tendon. Gently push the tendon to the side to allow your thumb to go deep, where there's resistance; flex your wrist up and down until you sense the trigger point.	This is a great point for relieving any nerve pain of the forearm. It also helps calm the mind. It's a so-called heart point (in Chinese medicine = heart disharmony). It promotes feelings of safety because it regulates the heart, calms the mind, and clears the head. It also helps with insomnia and fear.
Back-Body Rest your hand with your fingers extended. Release left Back G with your right thumb and vice versa) in circular movements, going deeper each time.	This point is the gate to opening the large intestine; it helps with headache, hangover, and constipation.
H Front-Body Place your index finger on the most prominent part of your hipbone. Count four fingers flat toward the middle of your body and locate the tender area.	This point helps with perimenopausal issues and libido.
Back-Body With your index finger on your front hip bone, locate the most prominent part of your back hipbone with your thumb. Count four flat fingers down toward your buttocks and then use your thumb to locate the pressure point.	This point helps with lower back pain and premenstrual pain. It also helps with lymphatic drainage and improves bloodflow.
I Front-Body Measure halfway between your hip bone and the outer part of your knee.	This point helps encourage bloodflow and lymphatic drainage as well as relieve knee/thigh/muscle pain from running or driving long hours or low back pain from flat feet or wearing high heels.
Back-Body If you imagine a line between the back of the hip (close to Back H) at the back of the knee crease, the middle point on the line will be Back I point.	This point helps encourage bloodflow and lymphatic drainage as well as relieve knee pain, low back pain, and calf pain, especially when combined with Back H and J.

Table 6. **Working with Self-Healing Trigger Points** (*continued*)

TRIGGER POINTS	NOTES
J **Front-Body** This point is toward the outside at the top of the thigh.	This point relieves lower back pain, knee pain, and muscle tightness from flat feet or high heels.
Back-Body This point is halfway between the Achilles tendon and the crease of the knee, directly in the middle of the leg (on the midline)	This is a great point for relieving pain and stiffness of the lower back and for contraction of the calf; it also helps with piles/hemorrhoids and helps release inflammation.
K **Front-Body** On your inner thigh, move three fingers up from the kneecap.	This point helps release any bloodflow to the ovaries or uterus and relieves premenstrual swelling.
Back-Body Grip the ankle and apply firm pressure with your thumb in circular movements for five seconds; repeat until the tightness is removed.	This point helps with pelvic pain, lower back pain, menstrual cramps, and hip pain. Outside the ankle helps increase bloodflow to the ovaries. Inside the ankle helps the uterus.
L **Front-Body** Bend your knee to ninety degrees, and with the index finger of that side, feel the outside bone below your knee. Press between the dip at a point two fingers toward the front from the outside of the knee.	This point helps with edema and localized swelling of the limb. It also helps insomnia or sleep disturbance caused by heartburn from stomach heat, relieves bloatedness, clears heat from the stomach channel, and eases nausea and vomiting (balances/ harmonizes the stomach).
Back-Body Back L is located under the heel crease.	This point helps with sluggish intestines, constipation, and premenstrual tension. It also relieves lower back pain and improves circulation.

Table 6. **Working with Self-Healing Trigger Points** *(continued)*

TRIGGER POINTS	NOTES
M Front-Body Sit on a chair and bend your knee to your chest. Use your right thumb for the left foot and vice versa. You can also do this in bed at night. Apply firm pressure between the first (i.e., big) and second toes. Now count six fingers flat from the top of the nail of your big toe and apply pressure there.	This point helps relieve anger, frustration, irritability, anxiety, headache, thirst, and dream-disturbed sleep. This point helps with pain in the shoulder, upper back, and upper arm.
Back-Body This point is located underneath Front N, beneath your fourth and fifth toe.	This point helps with pain in the shoulder, upper back, and upper arms.
N Front-Body This point is between the fourth and fifth toes, two to three fingers up from the little toe, at the tendon when you flex your little toe.	This point helps with decision making and pain in the upper back and shoulder. When you are feeling self-doubt and overload, it calms the mind, clears the brain, and releases the gall bladder.
Back-Body Apply firm pressure on the sole of the foot with your thumb between the second and third toes, starting at the ball of the foot and moving toward the midline.	Practitioners of Chinese medicine believe that this point is the foundation of the yin and yang. This point calms the mind, helps with feelings of panic, and releases tension in the diaphragm to help breathing.
O Back-Body This point is located under the big toe.	The outside of the big toe helps with the neck and thyroid. The middle underside of the toe helps the hypothalamus deliver messages to the ovaries, encouraging libido and fertility. The inside helps with sore throat.

As you use these pressure points, say to yourself, "While I am applying pressure and I feel the pain or bruised area, I allow my body to release anger, frustration, heat, and inflammation. I forgive and let go of [name the person]'s actions, and I am fully alive. I move forward. I release anger." Breathe in, close your eyes, and feel the pain moving out of your muscles. Say, "I am balanced. I am grounded. I let go."

RELEASE-WEEK MORNING GLORY ENHANCEMENTS

Now we'll expand your Release program by adding a few elements to your Morning Glory routine. As noted earlier, I like to describe that routine as a daily reset; it's the way I get in touch with myself and get grounded before I go out into the world.

Release-Week Morning Glory Ritual at a Glance

- Warm water with lemon (except first three days—see "Positive Function" below)
- Tibetan Rites
- Breathing exercise
- Daily reflection
- Dry brushing
- Shower
- Self-massage with oil
- Nine-point meditation

Dry brushing.

After your daily reflection and before your shower, do a session of dry brushing. As I mentioned earlier, I've been doing this every day since I was a teenager, when my mom taught me this ancient practice. One form of dry brushing was invented in Greece—of course!—and it's long been a favorite grooming habit in Europe. With its seventeen square feet of surface area, skin is our largest cleansing organ, akin to our lungs and kidneys. When you dry-brush, you increase your circulation, shed dead skin cells, and stimulate lymphatic drainage, moving nutrients from your blood into your cells and removing toxins. Your lymphatic system, which is responsible for about 15 percent of your body's circulation, transports white blood cells that help rid the body of toxic materials. Even blockages on the surface of the skin can cause congestion throughout the lymph system, and dry brushing is one of the most effective ways to ensure that the system stays active and clear.[2] Another beautiful bonus: Brushing stimulates production of collagen and elastin fibers, which help support skin as it ages. (But please note: Never do dry brushing on your face; instead, use a wet, soft loofah with some facial cleanser.) I find that dry brushing wakes up my skin and my psyche in ways almost nothing else does!

Start with a brush specifically designed for dry brushing. Some people recommend vegetable-based brushes, but I love the boar's-hair brush that I bought in the United Kingdom. Unfortunately, boar's-hair brushes aren't as common in the States. (See appendix B for suggested brands of body brushes.)

Be warned: Your skin may be very sensitive to dry brushing at first, so go gently. Work the brush in circular movements, starting with the soles of your feet, working upward, and always in the direction of your heart. (When stimulating circulation and lymph system, you always want to be brushing in the direction of venous and lymphatic flow.) Proceed like this:

- Soles of feet

- Tops of feet

- Calves

- Thighs

Now move to the back. Remembering to brush in the direction of the heart, alternate sides, moving in this order:

- Buttocks

- Lower back

- Sides

- Lower abdomen

- Upper abdomen

- Chest

Figure 15. **Dry Brushing for Lymphatic Drainage**

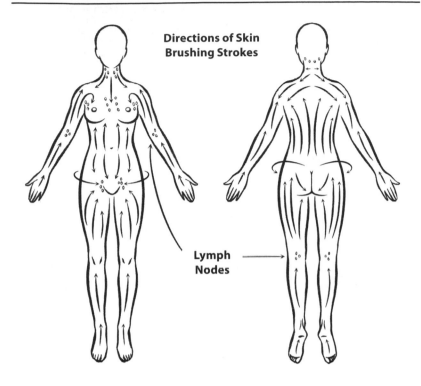

Stop there, and then start on your arms:

- Fingers

- Palms

- Backs of hands

- Forearms

- Elbows

- Upper arms

Once you're done, your skin should feel soft and alive and ready for your shower. Take one last look in the mirror and thank your skin for breathing and your heart for beating. Then take your shower as normal.

At the end of your shower, as the water runs off your body, say a silent prayer:

> I am starting to take control of my body, my mind, and my emotions. I am starting to clean myself up. I am watching my fears and my anxieties wash away. I am the power and authority. I am taking control of my body. I am taking control of my life, my fears, my insecurities, and my guilt—all those things that create pain in my life.

Now visualize all the negative feelings, having been washed from you, circling down the drain. Get out of the shower and do your self-massage with oil as usual.

Nine-point meditation.

When you're done with your self-massage with oil, it's time to transition to your morning meditation. The Release-week version is slightly more involved than the morning meditation you did in the Reflect stage:

Prepare your special place. Light up your incense and candle; let the smell of the smoke prepare your senses. Clear the room to allow light and positive energy to flow around you. Apply some calming, soothing lavender oil to protect and ground you. Place nine drops on your skin, one drop on each of these areas:

- Your forehead, between your eyebrows

- The back of your neck

- Your heart area

- Your throat

- The bottom of each foot

- Your lower back/sacrum area

- The inside of each wrist

With the drops in place, lie down on your back with your arms at your sides, your palms up. Close your eyes and take three breaths in and out, slowly and deeply, to the bottom of your lungs. Close your mouth and breathe through your nose. In your mind's eye, connect each of the points of oil together: Trace one breath from the bottom of your feet, going up your lower back, and then up to your neck. Then take another breath from those special oil points on your wrists, to your heart, to your throat. Say to yourself the following words (or a personalized version that hits the same notes):

> I am here today to free my mind from pain and fear. I am happy where I am today. I take a deep breath in and allow my breath to be louder than my thoughts. I say to those thoughts that would hurt me, "Stop playing games with me; stop taking me to that negative place. Leave my body."
>
> I am here today to allow my in-breath to help me understand. I am present; I am safe; I am alive; I am happy; I am back in my body. I am in the positive and I do not allow my fear to scare me.

When you take a deep breath in, you bring attention to your thoughts, fill up your "tank." When you breathe out, you release your pain, release your fear. Deep breathing stimulates a pronounced physiological response: Your heart rate and blood pressure slow, your parasympathetic nervous system activity increases, and you feel invigorated and alert.[3] That classic advice to "slow down and take a deep breath" continues to be an excellent guideline in all situations, especially those of high emotions.

With the addition of dry brushing and the nine-point meditation to your Morning Glory ritual, you'll have an even greater Release experience first thing in the morning.

SALT-AND-PEPPER BATH

Every time you take your shower in the morning, you're using the Morning Glory ritual to help you visualize your negative energy flowing down the drain. Now I want to talk about another therapeutic use of bathing: a bath with salt and black pepper.

This bath helps relieve pain and inflammation in your muscles—and it also has a healing effect on your mind. A ten-minute bath after work or late in the day can press the RESET button and allow you to be fully present with your family in the evening. A research review article in the journal *Current Directions in Psychological Science* found that washing your hands or taking a shower can help you release feelings such as doubt, regret, or a sense of being morally wrong. The researchers believe that this mechanism might be one we evolved with, to help drive early humans to remove contaminants; alternatively, it might simply be that we humans like to link abstract thoughts ("I had a hard day") with direct sensory experiences ("I'll wash it all off in the bath").[4] If you think about how many religious and spiritual rituals involve bathing (e.g., baptism with holy water), it makes sense that water would have an association with purification and a fresh start.

As soon as you arrive home from work or after a busy day at home, start the bath—as hot as you can stand it—and add two cups of Epsom salts and three to five drops of aromatherapy black pepper oil. Because Epsom salts are made of magnesium sulfate, they help your body to absorb magnesium, which helps to balance out your calcium levels and support the health of your parathyroid gland. Epsom salts also help with bloating, stiffness, or soreness.

As the bath is filling up, take a few minutes to tidy up or get kids started on homework. Then, while everyone else is occupied, sink into the tub and, like a child who's been playing in the mud, wash away the "dirt" from your day. Whether it was your negative colleagues or your boss, all visions of others' angry body language can be washed away, too. (Alternatively, you can do this in the steam room or in the shower at the gym.)

During the rough and tumble of our day, it's easy to lose ourselves. The following meditation is a vital part of the cleansing ritual and allows for both grounding/resetting and self-compassion. Close your eyes and see a white light or a white sheet protecting you. Take a moment to think this silent meditation:

I will let go. I will move forward.

This exercise is especially important for mothers who run around and serve everyone else's needs without properly attending to their own. In fact, it's *mandatory* for those women. (Trust me: I know your excuses. Just make it happen.)

If you have a more intense weight pressing down on you, one that you may have taken out on an unsuspecting, undeserving loved one, this is an ideal time to give yourself a pass, too:

> I am in pain, upset about _____, so I took it out
> on _____. I have to let go, let it leave my body. I get rid
> of the negative: Dirt, go away; leave me alone. I release my
> negative thoughts. I forgive my actions and move forward. I am
> safe; I am protected. I am healthy. I am strong. I am free from
> emotional drainage. The pain is leaving my body.

Then think of your kids, your spouse, a dear friend—anyone who makes your whole body smile and gives you "happy wings." Think to yourself:

> Thank you for your love. Thank you for your light. Thank you
> for letting me be me. I am so grateful for you.

(As with all the meditations in this book, please feel free to modify them to suit your circumstances, but try to stick with the core intention. Here, that intention is "letting go.")

Hold yourself to a short bath. Just ten minutes will be miraculous, you'll see. My reasoning? If you make it short, you'll be more likely to do it more often—which will help you more than doing a forty-five-minute bath once a month (or year).

DAILY NAP

By now, you've entirely shifted your attitude and approach toward sleep, right? You've been following all the suggestions from the Reflect chapter, so you start each day armed with seven to eight hours of solid, nourishing sleep. If that's *not* the case, I understand; I know how hard it can be to get yourself to sleep at a reasonable hour and allow your body the time to wake up naturally. Sometimes it just doesn't seem possible. If you're getting insufficient sleep, you can make up for it with a lovely, peaceful, restorative nap.

I can think of no more relaxing, luxurious, self-soothing way of releasing during your busy day. I squeeze in a quick nap (or at least a lie-down) almost every day. It helps me be a better mom, wife, healer, and overall human being. After pulling down the shades, I put a cloth over my eyes, let go of all the pressures, and tune out for twenty to thirty minutes.

According to Sara Mednick, an assistant adjunct professor of psychiatry at the University of California, San Diego, and coauthor of *Take a Nap! Change Your Life,* napping boasts many scientifically proven benefits:

- Boosts your mood

- Stimulates your creativity

- Sharpens your memory

- Decreases your stress

- Increases your alertness

- Speeds up your motor performance

- Cuts your risk of diabetes, heart attack, and stroke

- Helps you lose weight

- Enhances your sex life

- Improves your perception, stamina, motor skills, and accuracy

- Improves your decision-making ability

- Diminishes your cravings for fatty, sugary foods

- Cuts your need for caffeine and other stimulants

- Improves your body's ability to regenerate skin and tissue

- Increases your levels of anti-aging growth hormone

- Keeps you looking younger

Miraculous, huh? In other cultures, naps are considered a normal part of the business day—yet taking a nap in the United States is somehow synonymous with being a child. Start with one or two naps this week. There's no perfect time; just choose a time that fits your schedule and your energy level. Some enlightened workplaces have a quiet room where you can escape for fifteen minutes of shut-eye. If yours doesn't and you work in a safe area, spend a few minutes dozing in your car or on a blanket in the park. If weekday naps seem absolutely ludicrous to you, stick with weekend naps for now—but both days. And if you have kids, you have the perfect setup: Surrender to the deliciousness of a nap with your kids— you'll all love it and you'll get an oxytocin boost from cuddling to boot.

With these new structure practices in place during the Release stage, you've given your body more chances to downshift, calming your nervous system. Now let's dive into the meat of the Release week: letting go of toxic foods.

Positive Function

You know by now that many of our problems with pain—not to mention overweight and chronic disease—are due to inflammation. And I firmly believe that inflammation itself is primarily caused by the large quantities of sugar and wheat we ingest in the U.S. diet.

I've designed the Release Meal Plan for maximum detoxification. During the Radiate week and beyond, you'll have a wider range of food options. (For a meal-by-meal breakdown of these Positive Feedback Meal Plans, please see chapter 7.) For best results, follow the initial cleansing regimen for seven days. On the Release plan, you're going to delight in fresh, delicious, whole foods such as a spinach salad with eggs and pomegranate seeds. Even more important than adding such foods to your diet is releasing those that have been affecting you in detrimental ways for years. In this chapter, I'll focus the discussion primarily on the foods that you need to *release*—the things you eat that make pain worse. In chapter 6—"Week 3: Radiate"—I'll speak at length about the delicious anti-inflammatory, pain-relieving, beauty-restoring foods that you'll be eating in their place.

Heavily processed foods (including processed meats), trans fats, and sugars turn up the heat on the inflammation in your body. Refined white-flour foods are a national addiction. Pasta, white bread, white rice, bagels, pretzels, and pizza dough are among the starchy foods that trigger the release of excess inflammatory cytokines. Trans fats—found in hydrogenated oils, margarines, shortenings, and many processed foods—damage the cells in the lining of blood vessels, contributing to heart disease; furthermore, they've been proven to increase depression by 48 percent,[5] not to mention increasing irritability and aggression,[6] insulin resistance, and bad cholesterol.[7] Drinks and foods flavored with various types of added sugar (especially high-fructose corn syrup) cause the spikes in blood sugar and insulin that are well-established triggers for insulin resistance and metabolic syndrome. *All* such foods are inflammatory: You must begin to think of them as poisonous and, to the very best of your ability, eliminate them from your diet.

Remember that this isn't a diet program in the sense of weight loss; you're not specifically trying to lose weight by eating less. You're releasing your pain and your negative thoughts and emotions by not feeding your emotions toxins such as sugar. In addition to reducing pain-causing inflammation and releasing toxins from your body, getting rid of disease-promoting foods will lower your blood levels of insulin, a hormone that, in excess, can encourage fat accumulation, diabetes, and even cancer. And while it's not the objective of the Release plan, many of my patients are thrilled to lose up to five pounds in their Release week.

Getting rid of toxic food can be the first step toward releasing other toxins in your life, be they people, jobs, or unhealthy influences. Rooting out and tossing negative hidden sugars and other inflammatory poisons will help you feel free of pain, grounded, and able to make the right decisions for yourself. Your body knows when you're happy—and when you're miserable. And all of that information comes to you from processes in the gut.

It's also important to remember that weight gain is just one effect of giving in to food cravings. Those late-night binges not only add weight, but also affect your mood, keeping you stuck in the negative. And even more alarming, toxic foods eventually wreak havoc on your overall health.

A major part of our immune system—populated with over a thousand different species of "good" bacteria—is contained in the gut. Over one hundred trillion of these intestinal microbes do very important work in the body, controlling inflammation, protecting intestinal health, and boosting immunity. What we eat has an immediate impact on our neurons, our hormones, and our immune system, all because of our personal reactions to foods.

Some foods cause reactivity in many people; others rarely cause problems. Even when people dutifully steer clear of processed foods and simple carbs, however, they may still have food-related problems that are specific to their body. When people have an intolerance to certain foods, such as gluten or dairy, eating those foods can cause inflammation in the gut. This intestinal inflammation directly affects the entire body and eventually shows up in my office (or that of another health professional) as pain, especially lower back pain. Here are some common symptoms associated with inflammatory foods.

- Digestive upset (excess gas, abdominal pain)

- Hyperactivity (in children)

- Lethargy or irritability

- Loss of sleep due to pain

- Lower back pain

- Muscle and joint ache

- Skin sensitivies (such as eczema)

- Water retention (puffy face, ankles, fingers)

Look again through your Food Diary to see if your mood significantly altered between one meal and the next. If so, make a note of what you ate that day. Is there a pattern? Do you notice any specific symptoms from the list above that seem to come and go, such as bloating in your face, or aching in your neck or wrists, or swollen fingers, with specific foods?

If you notice that a specific type of food causes a negative response like those listed above, remove that food from your diet for the Release stage (even if it's in the Release Meal Plan), to test whether that food was causing the issue. For example, Virginia, a patient who was struggling with some extra pounds, really wanted to eat more vegetarian meals. But she found that whenever she ate mushrooms (a vegetarian staple), she felt off—her stomach would bloat and she would get a slight headache. Sure enough, when we did a full food sensitivity profile for her, we found that she had a sensitivity to mold—and mushrooms are a type of fungus. The problem was, her husband absolutely adored mushrooms; he wanted them for every meal. We tested her with various types of mushrooms and discovered that her reactivity was much more pronounced with certain kinds (including shiitake and portobello). Now Virginia eats those only very rarely; and, armed with this information, her husband now buys innocuous button mushrooms and modifies the way he prepares them.

When we get to the Radiate stage of the program, I'll show you how to test your sensitivity to a certain food by reintroducing it on a day that you eat only foods you know your body absorbs readily. Combined with the full list of Radiate foods, this information will help you build an eating plan that will work to keep you healthy and inflammation-free for the rest of your life.

Now it's time to begin your seven-day Release Meal Plan. Review the meal-by-meal breakdown in chapter 7 first and check out the shopping list in appendix C, to ensure that you have all the supplies necessary in the house. You may also want to rid your cupboards of *un*wanted supplies— those toxic sugars and starches you'll be avoiding. Some people prefer to get started on the eating program right away, and then do their kitchen cleanse; others prefer to toss out all the garbage first, and then begin the program with a clean slate. I leave that choice up to you. We'll begin here with the Liver Flush, the first element of the Release Meal Plan, but feel free to skip ahead a few pages, to the section titled "Release the Toxic Inflammatory Foods," if cleansing your kitchen *first* feels more natural to you.

RELEASE (DAYS 1–3): CLEANSE VIA A LIVER FLUSH

The Release Meal Plan begins with a three-day Liver Flush, as noted above. The aim of the Liver Flush is to cleanse the body and allow the immune system to heal. The cleanse, or detoxification, is an age-old process that's a part of many cultural and religious traditions. The premise is simple: When we stop eating for a significant period of time, the body has time to heal itself naturally. The amount and type of foods in the standard American diet overwhelm the body's resources and put us in a state of constant digestive processing. We're born with powerful self-healing capabilities, but for many us, the body literally doesn't have the time or energy to do the necessary healing work. With this liver cleanse, we provide the body the time and nutrients to flush out all the toxins and restore natural balance.

This is a fail-safe and important regulatory process. When my patients are in pain and showing some of the symptoms of toxic overload (such as extra weight gain, puffy eyes, irritability, blotchy skin), I advise them to just drink water and have no food for the remainder of the day. The next day, they inevitably feel much better. No medication necessary! The Liver Flush is designed as a more livable way to get that important cleansing done over a three-day period.

Before we turn to specifics of each meal during the Liver Flush, let's talk about water. The word "flush" implies water—and rightly so. You'll want to drink eight to ten glasses of water over the course of the day. (More on calculating the exact amount *you* should drink in a few pages.)

Breakfast.
During the three days of the Liver Flush, either eat no breakfast or wait one hour after rising before eating a smaller-than-usual portion of millet

or oats. (Having no breakfast increases the cleansing action, but it can be challenging for some people.) With either approach, you'll have enough nutrition and calories to get through your day, but the slight reduction in food and the alteration in the nutritional profile will mildly challenge your system and stimulate the Adaptive Response. In place of breakfast (or in addition to your oatmeal), have a Liver Flush Smoothie (recipe below).

Lunch and Dinner.

Feeding your body lighter meals is the only way to heal. The three-day period of the Liver Flush is a gift to your body and health. For these three days, your lunch and dinner should be limited to leafy vegetables, vegetable-based soups, and raw or lightly steamed vegetables, along with fruit. Eat baked sweet potatoes or squash and as much sprouted seeds and grains as possible: alfalfa, mung beans, black-eyed peas, and so on. Sprouted seeds, whole grains, and beans have high levels of fiber, protein, and antioxidants, as well as some digestive enzymes.

(Note: Once you're out of the Release week and into Radiate and beyond, you can bring back the Liver Flush whenever you're feeling bloated and in need of a little cleanse. Aim to eat soups and vegetables for two to three days to cleanse; then slowly introduce other foods over the next three to four days. You'll look clean and feel clean and lighter.)

Snacks and desserts.

Stick to fresh fruit, seeds, and nuts for snacks and treats during this period.

And don't forget: *Drink plenty of water!*

————————

Some of the most beneficial chemicals in vegetables and fruits—your main foods during the cleanse—evolved first as toxins to ward off insects and other predators; and these same chemicals activate an adaptive stress response in our cells. Certain phytochemicals, such as resveratrol (in red wine), sulforaphane (in garlic and onions), and curcumin (in curries and mustards), are thought to protect cells against injury and disease by stimulating antioxidant enzymes, growth factors that foster brain cell growth, and proteins that help cells withstand stress.[8]

By limiting the foods you eat during Release, both in type and quantity, you tap into your body's innate self-cleansing properties as well. New evidence suggests that sporadic fasting or food restriction can actually have a very therapeutic effect on your blood sugar and lipid profile, not to mention your weight.[9] Sporadically limiting your foods in this way may allow you to reap the same health benefits—fewer pounds, better blood sugar regulation, less inflammation and belly fat—as someone who restricts their calories every day.[10]

Your body is talking to you: Sometimes you need a good cleanse away from negative foods and people, some time and space to be alone. The three-day Liver Flush is an excellent opportunity to make time for yourself and turn down a few invites, spend the evenings in, and focus on rest and relaxation. (Also a good idea to stick a bit close to a toilet, just in case the Liver Flush decides to "flush" a bit more suddenly than normal.)

The Liver Flush will help rid your body not just of food toxins but of emotional toxins as well. Often before people start the Positive Feedback program, they feel a tremendous amount of unresolved anger; as a result, they feel hot and sweaty, and they shout all the time. The Liver Flush will help you focus, forgive, and let go of anger.

Liver Flush Smoothie

Mix in a blender:

Juice of 1 grapefruit
Juice of 1 lemon
½ cup olive oil
1 clove garlic
2 to 3 slices ginger

Every ingredient in the Liver Flush Smoothie has its own anti-inflammatory power:

- Grapefruit has lycopene, an antioxidant that can tamp down inflammation.

- Lemon has numerous anti-inflammatory actions (see "The Beauty of Lemon," below).

- Extra-virgin olive oil contains a recently discovered antioxidant called oleocanthal, which has anti-inflammatory properties similar to ibuprofen.[11]

- Garlic contains sulfur compounds that help the liver with detoxifying.

- Ginger, a potent anti-inflammatory and blood thinner, protects the liver by preventing cholesterol absorption.

Drink the Liver Flush Smoothie first thing in the morning, right after your Morning Glory warm water with lemon. Follow with another large glass of water. Then finish the rest of the Morning Glory ritual. Follow that (during these Liver Flush days) with a cup of hot water or hot liver-cleansing tea. During the day, continue to drink as many cups of such tea as desired:

- Fennel tea

- Nettle tea

- Peppermint-leaf tea

- Anise tea

- Green tea or jasmine tea

You may add lemon to these, but try to avoid honey until after the cleanse.

RELEASE (DAYS 1–7): FALL IN LOVE WITH LIQUIDS

In this Release week, as mentioned, fluids are crucial. You should drink at least eight to ten glasses of water and/or herbal tea daily, in addition to your smoothies. I have a portable water bottle that I carry with me all

The Beauty of Lemon

What you eat is what you are. While you're releasing negative foods from your diet, you're helping yourself let go of the negative. An effective way to speed this process of cleansing your system is to drink plenty of lemon water. In addition to your warm water with lemon during the morning, consider infusing every glass of water you drink with a slice or two of fresh lemon. Lemon's aromatherapy power helps stimulate sharp thinking and wakefulness. In addition, delightfully, lemon helps release toxins and clean you out in many ways. Lemon has the following benefits:

It's an alkaline-booster, for better pH balance to counter inflammation.

It contains antioxidants to fight cancer-causing free radicals.

It serves as a digestion aid.

It's a diuretic to temper puffiness.

It's an immune system supporter.

It's an iron-absorption booster.

It's a liver cleanser.

It contains a prebiotic (pectin, contained in the white flesh under the skin).

It's rich in vitamin C, to counteract cortisol and stimulate synthesis of collagen.

---

day—I call it "my pink friend." I use it for smoothies in the morning and nettle tea the rest of the day. I fill it up with water for hikes. Basically, it never leaves my side.

Be sure to drink only filtered water—no tap water. The Environmental Working Group, a nonprofit organization devoted to environmental and public health, has identified 316 chemicals in U.S. tap water, 202 of which are not regulated. If you can afford it, have a reverse osmosis filter installed in your house. It's the absolute gold standard, but it's expensive. Otherwise, a carbon filter pitcher—such as a Brita—will filter out most contaminants for a very reasonable price.

With the Release plan, you'll be making a smoothie every single day. After you've completed the first three days, you can begin to branch out into different smoothies. I use the NutriBullet, a nutrition extractor/ pulverizer: It allows me to throw in the entire fruit (seeds and all), so I don't miss a drop of fiber or other nutrients. (See additional smoothie recipes in table 12, found in chapter 7, and a list of smoothie powders in appendix B.) Some of my favorite smoothie ingredients (goat's-milk yogurt, pineapple, almonds or protein powder, flaxseed, banana, blueberries, kiwi, and a spoonful of olive oil) have all-star anti-inflammatory properties—as well as a bunch of other health benefits. For example:

- **Pineapple:** We now know that pineapple, long considered a no-no because of its high sugar content, is one of the strongest anti-inflammatory fruits on the planet. It also has bromelain, a digestive enzyme that helps the body digest protein.

- **Flaxseed:** A vegetarian source of anti-inflammatory omega-3s, flaxseed also helps increase energy, boost mood, and relieve pain, as well as ease digestion.

- **Sea buckthorn:** The oil of the sea buckthorn has a lot of good omega fats that help lower cholesterol and triglycerides. Sea buckthorn also helps to balance the production of gastric acids in a way that reduces inflammation and strengthens the immune system. Other antioxidants in sea buckthorn protect cells from free radicals and damage caused by excess sun, pollutants in the environment, smoking, and drinking.[12]

RELEASE (DAYS 1–7):
RELEASE THE TOXIC INFLAMMATORY FOODS

Now for the "release" of Release week: It's time to get rid of all foods that feed your negative. Start reading the back of every box or bottle you eat or drink from, and be skeptical of long ingredient lists. Shoot for five ingredients or fewer—all words that you recognize, without scary suffixes—and avoid sugars and derivations of sugar. Sugar lurks, hidden, in many products. For example, I was really surprised to see how much sugar was in my beloved almond milk. It wasn't "pure"; it was full of sugar.

Go through your cupboards and gather up all candy, all cereals, all cake mixes. Even if they're gluten-free, they can be full of sugar. Pile all the garbage foods on the table and then dump each, one at a time, into the trash, saying goodbye. Ditch the following:

Artificial creamers

Artificial sweeteners

Bagels, white flour (and products made from it), and wheat bread

Cashew nuts, salty nuts, pistachios, peanuts, Brazil nuts

Coffee in excess (more than two cups per day)

Cow's milk, as well as cheese and yogurt made from cow's milk

Eggplant

Energy drinks

Fast foods

Gluten-based products (wheat, oats, rye, and barley)

Ketchup

Margarine

Mayonnaise

Mushrooms, especially shiitake

Oranges, tangerines

Pickles

Processed meats (bacon, ham, pork, hot dogs, sausages)

Soy beans, soy sauce, any processed soy product

Spicy foods, chili powder

Spirits, such as vodka and whiskey

Sugar, candy

Sugary cereals, granola, corn flakes

Tomatoes, tomato juice

Vinegar, all types

White potatoes

Now let's talk about a few particularly troublesome categories of food: wheat, dairy, red meat, and sodas.

Wheat.

While refined wheat products are the most inflammatory, wheat itself— even whole grains—can cause problems, because of its high volume of gluten, a type of protein that gives bread its stretchiness. If your reactions to gluten are strong, go to an allergist with expertise in food sensitivities to have yourself tested; he or she will let you know if you have an intolerance or a full-blown allergy. Banning all gluten would be a challenge— indeed, some foods I recommend, such as rolled oats, have gluten. That said, I do believe that striving to reduce wheat products can help minimize inflammation. The findings of a recent animal study published in the journal *Immunology* suggest that gluten can increase inflammatory cytokines even among those who don't have an intolerance or allergy.[13]

Dairy and red meat.

Most of us were raised to believe that full-fat dairy and red meat were bad for us because of the saturated fat and cholesterol. Then the low-carb craze came along and refuted that, claiming that meat was not only not bad for you, it was vastly preferable to the blood-sugar-increasing nonfat foods we'd been eating instead (pasta, air-popped popcorn, salads with fat-free dressing).

Now researchers are discovering that there is in fact an increased heart attack risk borne by meat-eaters, but that risk doesn't come from the meat itself; it comes from a chemical that's triggered by bacteria that live in the digestive tract only of meat-eaters. Vegetarians and vegans don't release this chemical, but meat-eaters do. Researchers believe that this chemical (known as TMAO, an acronym for its chemical structure) allows cholesterol to work its way into artery walls, stiffening them and causing arteriosclerosis, as well as preventing the body from releasing extra, unneeded cholesterol. This is no joke, because researchers believe that a raised TMAO level increases the risk of heart attack without even taking into account any of the traditional risk factors, such as smoking, high cholesterol, and high blood pressure.[14]

Much in the same way, dairy can harm the good bacteria balance in the gut. A study published in the journal *Nature* found that a diet high in dairy saturated fats helped host a harmful microbe called *Bilophila wadsworthia,* often found in people who have inflammation in their intestines.[15] The researchers believe that these dairy fats change the composition of the bile, which in turn changes the composition of the good-to-bad bug ratio in the gut. As the balance shifts, it can trigger an immune response that increases inflammation. Indeed, this is thought to be a very common reaction among adults.

So, if dairy fats are bad, what about skim milk? Well, I believe nonfat dairy may even be a bit worse, as the high lactose content raises blood sugar in the absence of any tempering fats—which can lead to more eating. While the milk fat in a cup of whole milk or even 2% may sate your hunger, the high glycemic index of a glass of fat-free milk makes it essentially no better for inflammation than a glass of sugar water.

That's why, while you're in the Release week, you won't have any red meat or dairy. When you get to the Radiate stage, you'll be able to enjoy red meat in moderation, because our brains and our muscles need a bit of red meat *once in a while*. But we absolutely need to get away from meat being the *centerpiece* of every meal—especially in a time of release.

Diet sodas.

And one final word about liquids: No more Diet Coke. No more Diet Pepsi. No more Diet Anything. No more soda, for that matter. Period. End of story.

Surveys have found that most people who drink diet soda drink more than twenty-six fluid ounces every day, which makes sense when you hear how many experts now believe that diet soda is addictive. I had a patient named Sara who was addicted to Diet Coke. She drank three liters a day (or roughly one hundred fluid ounces)! She refused to even consider making a change. During our Reflect work, we discovered that Sara's lower back pain stemmed from having felt abandoned by her mother during a messy divorce. She was fourteen at the time, and she felt responsible for the rift in some way, but she'd learned to bury her pain and anger.

Flash-forward a few years, and she married young and had three girls. She did everything she could for her family, unfortunately losing herself in the process. Her back pain had been going on for years when her husband finally sent her my way. After studying her Body Timeline and her Food Diary, she was able to identify the source. As we talked more, Sara began to see that diet soda was the fuel of her pain: She drank to get energy to be at the whim of her family. Once this light went on, she understood how and why she needed to make the change I'd been recommending. Today, she's kicked her diet soda addiction, her back pain is gone, and she's learned how to make time for herself again—without her reliance on soft drinks to keep her going.

A study of over 250 thousand people found that those who drank more than four cups of soda (especially diet) each day—thirty-two ounces— were 30 percent more likely to develop depression than those who drank no soda.[16] And those who think they're protecting their health by drinking soda with artificial sweeteners instead of sugar are sorely mistaken. Sucralose (Splenda) has been found to decrease insulin sensitivity by

20 percent.[17] Furthermore, a preliminary study presented at a prominent health conference suggested people who drink diet soda have a 61 percent higher chance of stroke and heart attack than those who don't.[18] I could go on, but . . .

Please, just stop!

REMEMBER: RELEASE CAN BE DIFFICULT

I always remind my patients: You might feel worse before you get better. Release is like going for a facial to get rid of blackheads when you've not had a facial in months. Your face will be clogged up, so you'll need a good exfoliation and a thorough cleanup—and you might look worse for a day until you start to shine and glow (and radiate!).

Instead of your normal bowel movement, you might experience some diarrhea or runny tummy, but don't worry—that's part of the cleanse. Let it go. Remember that all the negative toxins need to leave your body to help free your mind. You're releasing your negative thoughts and emotions by not feeding your emotions toxins such as sugar; you're releasing your negative food habits to prepare yourself for a big change in your

Surprising Spices

Food sensitivities and allergies can come from surprising sources. For example, according to allergists at the American College of Allergy, Asthma, and Immunology, 2 percent of all food allergies are to spices such as garlic and cinnamon.[19] Spice blends can contain up to eighteen spices, and the hotter the blend, the more likely an allergy can be triggered. Spices also appear in nonfood items, such as personal care products—body oil, moisturizer, toothpaste, perfume. Once you know you're sensitive to a spice, don't forget to check those personal care product labels.

life—a transformation. You're getting stronger so that you can make strong decisions for yourself.

You can help the action of the Release process by adding in a bit of peaceful movement. Let's consider what positive motion looks like on the Release program.

Positive Motion

If you've been doing your Tibetan Rites every morning, you've likely found that you can do more repetitions or hold the poses for a longer time by now. I'm not going to ask you to step it up or add any additional *strenuous* exercise during Release. Why? Because if you challenge yourself, you'll trigger your stress response, even if you don't intend to. Vigorous exercise increases the level of oxidative stress and inflammation in the body, and it can be especially taxing during a time of cleansing. So try not to do any intense exercise above and beyond your current level of fitness. Instead, simply keep your body moving in the course of your day, to encourage bloodflow and discourage your lymphatic system from becoming static. In this stage, for additional exercise, I recommend adding fifteen-minutes walks and gentle or restorative yoga.

TAKE A QUICK STROLL

A fifteen-minute walk won't increase inflammation but will have a drastic impact on your overall health. Squeeze as many of these short walks into your day as possible. I recommend three a day, one after each meal. A study published in the journal *Diabetes Care* found that a brief walk directly following a meal can help your body absorb the inevitable blood sugar spike from the meal and significantly improve your glycemic control. Indeed, the three walks—instead of just one, for forty-five minutes—were more effective at lowering glucose peaks after meals.[20] This is particularly important because those increases in post-meal glucose are one of most highly predictive risk factors for cardiovascular disease.[21] I love this approach because (a) you can do it anywhere on earth, at any time; (b) you can easily create a well-entrenched habit (after every meal, I walk!); (c) you'll see and interact more with your neighbors throughout the day (and we know how important social support is to overall health and vitality). I've also started to get my patients hooked on Jawbone, a diet- and exercise-tracking device that you can use to track steps walked, blood pressure, food intake, and even the number of hours of quality sleep you get.

DO SOME GENTLE YOGA

You may be very disciplined and love to work out, hard. Taking it easy may not come naturally to you. But please don't worry that you're not burning calories or building muscle this week. This stage isn't about that; it's about healing from your pain. It's also about changing your automatic stress response from one that's highly reactive to one that's more relaxed, steady, contemplative, and *not* quick to react.

If you're really eager to add more activity, do some gentle yoga. When you stretch and lengthen your body, when you hold a pose a bit longer than is entirely comfortable, you'll automatically activate your stress response. But here's the genius of yoga, the Adaptive Response at work: While you're challenging yourself, and thus engaging your sympathetic nervous system, you're also breathing deeply and deliberately, staying focused, and staying present in your body. In other words, you're actively engaging and training your parasympathetic nervous system to counterbalance your sympathetic nervous system. In this way, yoga strengthens the "cool" response of the parasympathetic system, training your brain to stop automatically sending your sympathetic nervous system into overdrive. It teaches you to approach any hectic or stressful experience in a calm, attentive state. And it also makes you feel fantastic.

Now let's move on to the Release work that can be the most challenging of all: emotion. If you've been carrying around a burden that has created pain in your life, it's time to let it go.

Quick Body Scan for Habitual Offenders

The deep work of the Reflect stage can sometimes distract us from more obvious sources of pain. As you're doing your Release work this week, take a quick body scan to ask yourself if your aches and pains could be caused by a simple habit you're doing (or not doing) in your daily life. For example:

Is my pain caused by something as simple as wearing the wrong shoes? Am I causing my own suffering by being stuck and just not moving forward—clinging to shoes (or relationships or jobs) that continue to cause me pain?

Is the culprit the heavy bag with books, files, and laptop that I carry every day to work—and the fact that I haven't stopped for a few minutes to clear my bag and clear my head and leave some things (including my worries) at the office?

Are my muscles aching because I spend my time in an overly air-conditioned office or home—which is causing them to seize? Am I simply tolerating my discomfort because I'm afraid to assert my rights to be comfortable?

Or is the problem my junky old mattress, which I don't value my health enough to replace because "I'm just too busy"?

Positive Emotion

You've emptied your literal cupboards; now it's time to throw open your emotional cupboards and see what's lurking in there, what thoughts and feelings are healthy and serving you, and what's not healthy, not serving you, and needs to be released. Now is the time to release all accumulated slights, pains, traumas—*whatever* is poisoning you—so that you can let go and move on.

Emotion work is probably the most important, and most challenging, of the entire Release week. I recommend that you space out the following activities over the week; don't do them all in one day. Release is an on-going process, one that may never be fully completed: Much like weeding a garden, you need to keep releasing, week after week, in order to access the luscious, life-sustaining harvest underneath the overgrowth. And if you keep facing your pain, you'll learn that it won't kill you. Simply put, the process of releasing gets better, easier.

RELEASE THE TIME-WASTERS ON YOUR TIME AUDIT

This exercise is an eye-opener that helps people finally make the connection between where they are and where they want to be. Give yourself an hour or so to do this audit revision and let it really sink in. The results will be worth it.

Get out your Time Audit from the Reflect stage and take a good hard look. Scan through the hours. Are there areas you can see where you know you've been killing time, not moving ahead? Are you spending too much of your life doing things that make you unhappy? Highlight all the hours in the audit spent doing tasks that *didn't* make you happy.

Now, here's the tricky part: Be honest. In your notebook, write out a reason that you do each of those particular unrewarding activities: Why do you think you're doing each?

Is it because you haven't found your passion yet? Something to drive you? Here's an example: Say you're afraid of being rude to your boring, nosy neighbor, so you drop everything when she stops by to chat. What if you were working on a project that consumed you—would you be more likely to say, "Sorry, can't talk now," or would you still feel beholden to be "nice" and continue a time-wasting conversation?

Perhaps you're still on that consumption track—you're consuming in-stead of producing. Do you think your life has value, that you're making a contribution to the world? Are you feeling powerless and lost? Or are you totally directed and know exactly why you're here and what your place is in the world—and those activities are part of "paying your dues" to get there? Where are these activities taking you?

Most of us in pain are running away in some fashion, trying to escape and therefore filling our lives with distractions. If this is case with you, it's time to let it go. Let it *all* go. Let go of the guilt. The regret. The self-torture. Each coulda-shoulda-woulda that keeps you from getting on with things and just moving forward. The huge, heavy baggage from former friends or lovers, or a less-than-supportive family. All of that, at this moment, exists only in your mind.

To support your letting go, take out a blank sheet of paper to supplement your Time Audit—and create a new schedule. Include all the stuff you did that you *enjoyed*—spending time with friends, reading a great book, exercising, cooking a delicious meal with fresh foods, even spending a lazy Sunday in bed. All the things that, when you did them, made you feel joy and satisfaction—even if they took only fifteen minutes.

Now, those spaces where you put crap television or endless web surfing or junk food binges or cocktail hours . . . those you scour. Wipe them clean. Pretend they're not even a possibility. Selectively take out unfulfilling tasks as well—those that you didn't *have* to do but did anyway.

In their place, write in the few things a week that you know would make a huge difference to your mental health. Walk at five thirty each morning with the dog? Put it in there. Meditation before bed? A session with your journal and a cup of coffee after the kids head for school?

Now look at this new schedule: This is where you *really* were. This is where your brain and your heart were while your body killed time. This is your true life.

Rather than waste your life in a dream world, zoned out from the things that really matter to you, start to think about your revised Time Audit as reflecting the true, real, actual events in your life—and the crossed-off events as mere hiccups that you'd like to soon forget. Switching your mind's orientation from "I'd love to do this" to "I *do* this" is a huge leap forward in terms of making something happen.

Make copies of this new schedule and hang it up throughout your house and your workplace. Tape a copy to your bathroom mirror, so you can read it during your Morning Glory ritual. Stick a copy in your purse or pocket. Stuff it into the visor in your car. Have this reminder around you all the time: *This* is my life. I may get distracted every once in a while, but this—*this* is where I really am. And then fake it 'til you make it!

RELEASE HARMFUL HABITS

Okay, I realize that simply walking away from unfulfilling activities is tricky. Those time-wasters that you *didn't* transfer over from your original Time Audit onto your ideal-world schedule are likely harmful, time-wasting *habits*. When we're hiding from our pain, running from it, we find lots of nice diversions to keep us from addressing it. While everyone needs a way to blow off steam and relax, sometimes these diversions can turn into addictions. It's not just drugs and alcohol we need to worry about: Many activities can be addictive, and can have equally devastating effects on otherwise productive lives.

How can you tell when your harmless distraction has turned the corner? According to the Stanton Peele Addiction Center in New Jersey, an addiction has five distinctive characteristics:[22]

1. You use it to erase negative feelings (such as pain, anxiety, or despair).

2. Using it detracts from other areas of your life (your job, friendships, or other interests).

3. It props up your wobbly self-image (you feel better when you use it; worse when you don't).

4. You organize your life around it (embedding it in firm routines).

5. You ultimately don't enjoy it; it becomes less and less enjoyable with time (yet you can't imagine not doing it).

What do you think—is there anything in your life that qualifies? Everything from smoking and gambling, to online shopping or porn, to fatty

foods and Internet use, to smart phones and social media, to tracking po-
litical news—any of these can be an addictive "substance." You'll know
you're ready to quit when you start to feel as though the benefit of the
addiction isn't worth the shame, the hassle, the money, or the time you're
wasting. The most successful "quitters" follow a very specific pattern:

1. They experience a building unhappiness and disillusionment.

2. They have a blinding epiphany: Eureka! This is bad for me! And
   I don't have to do it anymore!

3. They deliberately change their pattern to break the harmful
   habit.

4. They change their whole self-image to that of a person who
   doesn't do that addiction.

5. They tackle each relapse head-on and don't let it drag them back
   into Negative Feedback.

If you're ready, make a deliberate plan to break the chains of each
harmful habit. If you've got multiple habits to work on, you can't transform them all in a day—but you can *plan* your transformation. The most
important tool at your disposal: your attitude. No one can do this but
you; no one *will* do this but you. You have to show up and be there for
yourself—no one else can do the hard work for you.

If your addictions include any kind of chemical substance—
prescription drugs, street drugs, alcohol, tobacco—you need some extra
help. Your life could depend upon it. Please reach out to your family
doctor and just say those words: "I need help."

CALL IN REINFORCEMENTS

With major changes in the offing in your eating habits, your food shopping, and how you spend your discretionary time, you've got challenges
ahead. Why not call in reinforcements? Regardless of the habit or addictive behavior, we could *all* use a bit of help. Sometimes just reaching out
for a hand can help you wipe away some of the shame and self-blame. It's

likely that your friend can empathize with you. That empathetic connection is therapeutic in and of itself.

Here's an idea: Gather the list of foods you're trying to release and, instead of going out for dinner with a friend, invite her over. Tell her you have no time for hors d'oeuvres and alcohol; you need help. Can she come over while you're going through your kitchen to get rid of foods that increase heat, tiredness, inflammation, pain? Or help you gather up all your old, unwanted clothes, books, and other household items—the stuff that you think is "too good to throw out" but that drags down your energy. It's time to let it all go. Your friend could help you box it all up and drive it to Goodwill with you, and then take you for a nice green smoothie afterward.

Another way a friend can help is if *both* of you support *each other* in overcoming bad patterns and habits. A Korean study found that when coworkers joined a quit-smoking challenge and were offered a reward if *everyone* succeeded in quitting, their quit rates shot to 50 percent (versus the average 4 to 7 percent of those who go it alone)[23]—quite a difference in effectiveness!

If you can find a friend who is truly supportive and whom you trust completely, you can use this effective solution with almost any Release challenge—food, smoking, exercise, not calling an abusive ex, you name it. Set up the reward as something you both really want—a weekend away in the city or at a spa, or a night on the town without spouses or boyfriends, or buying a pair of high-end shoes you'd never buy just for yourself (but now that you're doing it for a friend . . .). Not only are you employing peer support ("C'mon, we can do this!"), you're also wielding a bit of peer pressure ("Don't mess up, because then neither of us gets a reward"). This approach can keep you accountable to each other and give you tremendous built-in cheerleading.

EXPLORE A NEW MODALITY

Another way you can look for help and support is to explore a new health modality. Before they come to me, many of my patients have been stuck in a health practitioner rut, falsely believing that all their mind-body health needs could be satisfied with one type of healing modality. Perhaps massage, maybe acupuncture, possibly Reiki. I guess it's my osteopathic background, but I find I'm never satisfied with just one approach to healing. I know that every person's energy is different, and every single day is different. You may have a health challenge one day that your acupuncturist would never be able to find—but a reflexologist could pinpoint right away.

I wish the United States had more European-type osteopaths, because I love the flexibility I'm able to use with my patients in the UK and other parts of the world. (Perhaps the closest parallels in the States are naturopathic doctors, but they're not very common.) During any session, I find the exact right combination that works for that person. Just doing cranial sacral therapy without the acupuncture for this person, or the manipulation or reflexology for that person, would seem incomplete. I think of myself as being like a carpenter—I have many different types of tools to help me help my patients. Or like a cook hovering over a pot of soup: a little more salt, a bit more pepper. I see what each person needs at any particular moment and I use that tool.

I've never done *just* massage without acupuncture or cranial work because I feel it's not grounding enough. Massage can release endorphins and natural opiates that help fight pain and help reduce anxiety and stress; it's great in that way. Yet I need to find the energy that's blocked and actually fix the blockage, get the nerves and blood supply and cerebral spinal fluid flowing, to get the glymphatic system working and allow everything to move along. That helps me feel that *my* part is complete, and now the person is able to go and do his or her work. The combination of these various therapies helps give both immediate and long-term relief.

While some naturopathic doctors in the United States use multiple modalities within each session, chances are you'll have to create this kind of experience for yourself. Rather than get locked into a rut with one type of practitioner, schedule an appointment with someone who practices a different type of healing modality, something you've never tried before. I know that some of these treatments are pricey, but one session can go a long way. Save up and splurge. I know you'll find it both eye-opening and valuable. Please consider one of these:

- Acupuncturist

- Chiropractor

- EMDR therapist (see page 164)

- Holistic nutritionist

- Hynotherapist

- Massage therapist (especially one skilled in neuromuscular and trigger-point therapy, lymphatic drainage, and cranial sacral therapy, for glymphatic release)

- Naturopathic doctor

- Reflexologist

Whether you seek the help of any other healing professional, I want you to do this: Believe in yourself. The most important professional advice I can give is to find someone you can trust who will locate your pain, who believes that the pain exists, and who cares about removing this pain. You want someone who is patient-centered, not doctor-centered.

It upsets me greatly that some professionals underestimate their patients' pain—or perhaps they don't specialize in pain so they don't understand how deep it can go. Or, even worse: They put fear in patients where none needs to exist.

I had a patient who was thinking of having a child. She went to her doctor complaining of pain in her lower back and ovaries. She had lost some weight and was tired, thinking about her next big job. Her doctor said, "Well, your eggs are aging and I'm not sure it looks happy down there." This woman was a dynamic, healthy thirty-eight-year-old. She and her husband had just started trying to get pregnant, and her doctor was already pushing her to do in vitro fertilization ("because it's guaranteed").

Wow. Does that sound like a healer?

When she came to me, I took a different approach. "Maybe the lower back pain is a message," I gently said. "Maybe it's urging you to stop and think, 'Hang on a second—my lower back is stiff, I'm overworking, and it's time to stop and think about my future.' You need to give yourself some rest, heal your pain, and send your ovaries some love, blood supply, and circulation so your eggs can be happy." She needed to give her sympathetic nervous system a break so that her body could recognize that she wasn't in crisis and that it was safe to make a baby.

Pain was the signal to make that change—and her doctor should have been the one to help her stop making excuses for the lower back pain and take steps to heal herself, instead of piling on pharmaceuticals and procedures to mask the underlying problem.

I'm always stunned when I hear these stories about uncompassionate, disconnected doctors or therapists. You deserve to be treated by a *healer,* not a drug-pusher or a pacifier. Keep looking for the right person to help you, someone who will take the time to listen to your pain and ask about all your symptoms. Someone who trusts your experience, who believes you when you speak about the intensity of your pain—because pain is whatever the person experiencing the pain says it is, not what the doctor thinks. I'd like you to find someone who believes and can help you understand that though the pain may be present now, it not only can be "managed," it can be released.

CREATE YOUR OWN RELEASE MEDITATION/VISUALIZATION

As I noted earlier, keeping a clear mental space is important to the work I do with clients. I always do a cleansing prayer (removing the "evil eye") on my way to clients. This meditation helps to reconnect me with my Greek heritage and helps me feel clear; it's important because it sets me up for a clean start in every session, no matter how challenging my prior client was.

An Answer to "Little t" Traumas: EMDR

If your traumas are still painful or raw, or if you feel like you could use some support through this Reflect * Release * Radiate process, I encourage you to reach out to a therapist, licensed clinical social worker, psychologist, or psychiatrist. Having a professional guide as you work through your pain could be the difference for you between checking out again and losing touch with your pain—and finally turning to face it, acknowledge it, and release it.

One therapy that I'm extremely impressed with, one that I hope will continue to expand and have broader application, is known as EMDR: eye movement desensitization and reprocessing. EMDR is a perfect example of how you can tap into your body's own internal self-healing mechanisms to bring you back into Positive Feedback.

First a bit of background. When you encounter a stressful experience, your brain needs time to process and "digest" that experience. After a fight with a friend, you might talk to other friends about it, journal about it, or simply sleep on it, possibly dreaming about it during the REM (rapid eye movement) phase of sleep. The next day, you probably feel better: Your brain has digested the experience and filed it away in the appropriate place in your memory; you can move on.

However, with some traumatic experiences, that process may go off track and the memories get misfiled, as it were. Those misfiled memories can then cause unconscious, automatic reactions to other events that may not seem related to an outside eye. Let's say your dad forgot to pick you up from dance class once when you were eight, and you stood there alone for a long time before the problem got sorted out. You may forever after be anxious when you're waiting for a bus or a plane, gripped by the fear that it will leave without you. But you may never connect this recurring fear back to waiting in front of the dance academy as a child.

All those memories are locked into the neural pathways in our brain as well as in nerves and muscle cells throughout our bodies. Research from the University of Texas suggests that victims of rape and sexual assault suffer mightily throughout their lives in eleven areas of psychological and social functioning,[24] including debilitatingly low self-esteem and fear of romantic intimacy. EMDR helps to release those traumas and let them go.

How does EMDR work? At the start of the eight-phase treatment, you and your therapist select a negative thought or image to target. During "processing," your therapist directs you to think about the memory and you move your eyes back and forth across your field of vision for twenty to thirty seconds, following the movement of the therapist's finger (or a stick or light, or even auditory tones through headphones). The theory is that by alternately stimulating both sides of the brain while the memory is evoked, EMDR triggers neurological and physiological changes that target several areas of your memory network.

The therapist talks you through the painful memory, using a stimulation sequence that allows the brain to properly process the memory of the trauma. Your brain "files" the memory correctly and you work with the therapist to replace the negative thought pattern associated with the memory with a positive one. As you move forward in therapy, you'll revisit the memory to test if you've truly digested it, and continue to locate other, related memories, digesting them in the here and now, and correctly filing them for the future.

Until a few years ago, EMDR had been used only in cases of severe trauma. Studies have shown that in as few as three sessions it can be tremendously effective at helping soldiers suffering from post-traumatic stress disorder and women who've been raped.[25] (The entire process takes up to eight distinct stages, but the sessions actively targeting the traumatic memory can be very few.) Recently, more and more mental health professionals are starting to use this important approach in their practice to help people who've experienced "small t" traumas: bullying, exclusion, relational aggression—things that are tremendously painful but aren't typically seen as major traumas.

While such events may not seem "major" to others, I've seen again and again how damaging these childhood slights and "small t" traumas can be; I see the aftermath with my patients every day. And many people I've talked with report that old, frustrating patterns of self-sabotage, anger, or anxiety that have resisted any change for years are suddenly resolved with a few sessions of EMDR. They're able to release painful memories that have been holding them back—simply let them go and move on.

If you believe that there's a trauma from your past holding you back, I urge you to investigate EMDR. Check out appendix B for a tool that will help you locate a practitioner in your area.

One of the most powerful focuses for meditations/visualizations in Release work is forgiveness. You can make your meditation/visualization as specific to your situation as you'd like.

Here's a critical point: You need to *feel* the insecurity or fear of the original offense in order to release it. If you don't engage with that emotion, and you don't release it, you'll continue to allow fear to get to you— you're only standing in your own way. You need to cut the cord with fear from the past so that you can truly live in your present life without allowing old patterns to take over.

Below is a meditation I wrote for a client who was going through a particularly challenging time in her marriage. Forgiveness is a scary thing— not for wimps! Your meditation practice is there to help you cope with your fears and overcome them.

I am here today to acknowledge my pain and my fear. I welcome my fear. I am strong. I am not scared. I am not alone. I can talk to my fear.

I am here today to forgive and love my father, who created that fear and abandoned me. I stop that fragile, vulnerable fear from the past, and I stop feeling punished.

I forgive my father, and I forgive myself for punishing myself and punishing my man.

I stop living in the past, in the negative.

I am taking a deep breath. . . . I am not alone. I am safe.

I do not fear the past and I do not allow anyone to put fear in me. I am present. I am grounded in this special moment. I am not taken from the past. I live in the positive. I do not go back to the past. I forgive. . . . I let go of living in pain.

I release any misunderstanding I still have. I release my fear, my anger. I am capable of great change. I am grateful for my journey and my childhood and my life. I am grateful for my children, my husband, all of our blessings, our health, our safety, and love for each other.

Take a moment to write your own forgiveness meditation in your notebook. What words would be most healing to you? Which relationships do you want to heal, at least in your own mind? Write down your meditation in the style you see above: "I am capable," "I am grateful," "I am safe."

RELEASE YOUR PAST VIA RITUAL

You've come to the end of the Release week, and you've done a lot of hard work. Congratulate yourself and mark the occasion with a cleansing ritual that will help you forgive yourself and others and release your past.

Think of every major religion—they all have a moment where you atone for your sins and forgive yourself and others for sins against you. Greeks, for example, have a fast for Easter week: We avoid dairy, meat, even olive oil for Lent. In Muslim cultures, for Ramadan, people fast, eating only during the evening hours. This week, you're doing something similar: cleansing your mind and body as if that process were a prayer for yourself, a cleanse for forgiveness.

Whenever you're ready for a big change in life, a transformation, you need to ready the ground, clear the space, and prepare yourself for what comes next. You need to be ready to make strong decisions for yourself. "I am doing this for myself. I am giving forgiveness to ___ ____ [Mom/Dad/ex-boyfriend/teacher/friend]. I am allowing myself to take charge."

Finding an appropriate ritual is a bit challenging for some people, especially if they've only just realized the source of their pain. One fairly universally helpful ritual is to select from your Body Timeline one of the most traumatic events of your young life and write a letter to your younger self explaining why that bad thing was not your fault. This exercise is about forgiving yourself. A forgiveness letter is also a potent tool when its forgiveness targets someone else (even if the letter is never sent).

I've known Alexandra, one of my clients, for almost ten years, but only recently did she confess a horrible story about her childhood to me. I knew that Alex was estranged from her entire family, but I never knew why. Then she wrote a forgiveness letter and shared that letter with me.

Turns out that when Alex thinks about her life as a young girl in Switzerland, she mostly remembers being very scared, spending a lot of time with her older sister alone in their big house. Their parents were always off doing something, so the girls had only each other. Neither one of them felt safe, because their father, when he was around, was very abusive. He wouldn't tolerate any dissent or backtalk. This prohibition worked out fine, until the girls hit puberty and did the standard talking back—and were met with brutal force in return. They learned to share their teenage angst with their mother; their dad was too much of a wildcard.

When Alex's older sister went away to boarding school, Alex felt abandoned. Now she had no one to help her feel safe. One weekend her mother went away, and her father brought home his girlfriend—apparently not caring one whit what his teenage daughter would think of his infidelity. He handed her the equivalent of a hundred dollar bill and said, "Our secret, right?"

Alex struggled mightily with whether to tell her mother. Finally, she did—and she wasn't prepared for what came next.

"Who says?" her mother demanded. Alex was dumbfounded. "No, really—who says? Am I supposed to take *your* word for it?" Alex stuttered, trying to find the words to tell her mother how sad she was for her, and how sorry she was that she had to go through this. But her mother didn't want to hear it.

"You're a lying little bitch, Alex," her mother shouted uncharacteristically. "Go to your room."

Alex retreated. She curled up on her bed, listening to her mother and father talking conspiratorially downstairs, and cried.

"Can you *believe* what she said to me?" her mother said to her father. "She's just jealous—now that Natalie is gone, she doesn't have anyone to spend time with. She's trying to turn me against you." Alex could visualize her father faking his shock and giving her mother a convincing hug, while he scowled over her shoulder.

Sure enough, as soon as her mother left the house, Alex's dad bounded up the stairs and gave her a beating. He'd hit her before, but never with the fury and force of that day. Then he pulled her down to the basement and put her into the dog crate. "Well, so much for us being friends," he said, and left her there for an hour, releasing her just before her mother came home.

Alex was devastated. She had no idea what to do—so she called her sister. Natalie was in London, a world away from the nightmare unfolding at home. She listened and murmured with sympathy, but when they hung up the phone, Alex felt even more alone than before. Natalie wasn't coming back for her; her mother didn't believe her; and her father was a monster. She started to question whether there was any point to staying alive. That's when she started cutting.

Twenty years after this devastating trauma, Alex was still nursing her wounds. Her parents had long since divorced. Her sister had finished university and stayed in England. Alex was struggling with panic attacks, lower back pain, and blinding headaches. Stuck in the in-between, Alex wanted to let go of her past but felt that she couldn't. Surprisingly, the biggest source of anger for her was not her dad or her mom—but her sister. Deep in her heart, Alex felt that Natalie had abandoned her at the very moment she needed her most. And yet Alex also *rationally* knew that Natalie hadn't meant to abandon her—that it was simply her time to leave the house.

When Alex brought me the letter to read, I was moved both by her hurt and by her willingness to forgive. As we discussed the entire trauma, Alex realized that her letter should have been addressed not to her father or her mother (as she'd written it), but to her sister, to forgive her. This letter of forgiveness would never be mailed—but it would be healing to simply write these added words: "Dear sister, I once blamed you for leaving me here in hell—but I now see that you were a young girl too, and you had no power to stop what was happening at home. You didn't abandon me; you saved yourself. And now I want to follow in your footsteps." Alex poured out the entire experience in full detail, leaving nothing out, putting it all on the page. After twenty years of unconsciously harboring resentment, anger, and hurt at her sister, she finally expressed the feelings that had been trapping her in mourning and loneliness.

To make her forgiveness more concrete, I asked Alex to read the letter out loud to me. As she spoke, I could see the weight of her childhood literally lifting from hers shoulders; her entire posture changed. I brought out a bowl lined with mother-of-pearl and took it and a lighted candle over to the end table beside her chair. She reread the letter out loud, then held it to the candle. Through our tears, we watched the ashes drift down into the bowl.

Alex's note was very dramatic. Yours might be simpler. But regardless of the content, once you've written your forgiveness note, it's time to release the pain. Choose one of the Release rituals suggested below to help you feel and see the release with multiple senses. Choose a symbol of poor health to Release ceremonially. For example:

- Label a chipped plate or vase with a personal limitation you want to release, and then take it out to the street or back alley and smash it!

- Build a backyard sacrificial bonfire and toss in unwanted memorabilia.

- Write a forgiveness letter to your younger self on a piece of rice paper and float it down a stream.

- Box up the unwanted memorabilia and take it to Goodwill or your local homeless shelter.

Yes, of course it feels satisfying to smash a piece of crockery to vent your frustrations. But remember: Rituals have a magical power in and of themselves to help us feel in control, in touch with our feelings, and able to endure even in our darkest hour. There's a reason every culture on earth has a very specific method of burying their dead. A "proper burial" ritual signifies closure. Consider this exercise your trauma's "proper burial"—allow yourself to sink into the process of it and imbue each bit of pottery or each burning letter with as much significance as possible. Help the ritual help you.[26]

VISUALIZE FORGIVENESS AND RELEASE

To end this chapter, I want to share a very specific visualization that my mother used to do with me, to help me rid myself of negative energy. Before you do this (or any) visualization, focus on your breath going in and out of your nostrils. You can do this visualization in the morning after your workout, when you get home from work, or on a break at the office, sitting on a chair in a quiet area or room. Make sure your back is supported so that the flow of energy can open up your chakras, meridians, and energy paths.

Close your eyes and take three deep, slow breaths, in and out of your nose.

Start visualizing a point between your eyebrows (the "third eye point"). Feel the energy and the higher senses of your soul. Count back numbers from three to one, slowly counting each number three times ("three-three-three, two-two-two"). Then count back from ten to one.

Visualize a white light or a window in that third eye point. In that white space, imagine a place you have happy memories of from your childhood, or make up a place in your mind that's peaceful and calm. See yourself walking on the beach or at the top of a mountain.

Now bring yourself to visualize a mirror surrounded by a blue light to your right side. This light represents your dark side and negative feelings. Visualize all the things you hate and fear about yourself pouring into the mirror. Being sick. Being angry. Being drunk. Being tired. Living in fear. Living in pain. Figure out what you want to focus on, and then take a good look at yourself in that mirror. Say to yourself,

I am in pain. I fear death. I am lonely. I hate myself. I am _____.

Now visualize a big stone in your right hand and smash that glowing blue mirror until there's nothing left. The mirror doesn't exist—you can't see yourself anymore.

On your left side visualize a mirror shining with a golden-white light. Look at your reflection. Say to yourself,

I am beautiful. My dreams have come true. I am achieving all my goals. I have a strong and supple body. I am healthy. I am glowing. I am with my special man. My kids love me. I am alive. I am happy. I signed the deal / got the job / finished the project.

The trick is to see yourself in that new role so clearly that you never see the old image of yourself again. Think of this as "positive mind control"—

you have the power to change your entire perception of yourself with this visualization.

Count one, two, three, four, five—and open your eyes.

You are in your body. You are in your space.

Check-In: Are You Ready to Radiate?

Now that you're getting to the end of the Release week, you're probably feeling much lighter. Many of my patients are amazed at the change in their skin in just a few days on the Release program. Is it the Liver Flush? The Release Meal Plan in general? Is it the Self-Healing Trigger Points? The extra salt-and-pepper baths, or the dry brushing? I believe that *all* the Release elements are important, of course, but the function work and the emotion work are where you'll see the most long-lasting results. If you've not yet done the Release the Time-Wasters on Your Time Audit, Release Your Past via Ritual, and Visualize Forgiveness and Release exercises, please do them before you leave the Release stage. The insights you'll gain through those exercises can carry you for many years into your radiant future.

Now let's move into the third stage of the Positive Feedback program—the Radiate stage—and see what life has in store for you!

Week 3: Radiate

Tension is who you think you should be.
Relaxation is who you are.

—Chinese proverb

M elissa had had a number of tough years. She'd delivered four kids in the span of eight years, and nursed every one until they were two years old. Her husband had a big job, so they made an agreement early on in their marriage that he'd focus on his work and she'd focus on the children. She joyfully made the choice to forgo law school and dove headfirst into being a mom—while also doing all the entertaining, along with research and packing for relocations every few years, to help her husband scale to new heights in his corporation.

Finally, the youngest was in third grade and the oldest was starting to look at colleges. All the kids were incredibly self-sufficient—her earlier labors had paid off. Aside from the typical teenage bumps, it looked as though all the kids were heading for smooth transitions. More often than not, Melissa found herself alone at home in the afternoon, all the kids at school for activities, her friends working, her husband flying off somewhere to give another presentation to another CEO. She was still doing a full load of volunteering at school, but it was getting less and less fun—fewer days of reading to the kids in the classroom or chaperoning field trips, more time spent raising money or making bake-sale items or sewing costumes for school plays (all solitary, largely unrewarding, tasks).

For the first time in sixteen years, Melissa was looking around for more entertaining and rewarding things to do. Her day-to-day existence just wasn't as fun anymore. One thing on her often-forgotten list: Finally get the checkup, Pap smear, bone-density scan, and vitamin D level test she'd been putting off for . . . yikes, looks like it'd been a few years.

Her doctor visit was fine; her gynecologist visit, fine. Even her mammogram visit was quick and uneventful. "Geez, why didn't I do this a year or more ago?" she thought. Took much less energy than worrying about it. But when she received a voice-mail the next day, asking her to come back to the breast imaging center for a second scan, she got a little nervous.

That night, she couldn't sleep. All she could think was, "Why did I wait so long? What if I have cancer? How could I have been so stupid?" When she got up the next morning, she froze a smile on her face and went through the motions. When she got to the imaging center, a technician ushered her in for the second scan. "Any ideas?" Melissa asked brightly. No, the technician said; she couldn't say anything—the doctor would call her later.

The next three weeks passed in a blur. The calls went from bad to worse:

> "There seems to be a small spot, nothing serious. We'll do a needle biopsy."

> "We found something, but we can get it out. It'll be a really fast procedure: You won't even realize it's happening."

> "We took a few of the nodes, just to make sure. We'll run the tests and let you know what's next."

After that last call, Melissa found herself sleepwalking through her day. The kids knew what was going on, and even though they were scared, they babied her the way she'd nurtured them for years. Her husband had flown back into town for the surgery but was expected in Hong Kong for an international conference right afterward. *I can handle it. Don't worry—just go; I'll be fine.* So he went.

In the couple of days it took to get the node results back, Melissa had a lot of time to herself. She took out the Positive Feedback packet she'd started a few months earlier but never completed. As she lay in bed with ice packs under her arm, she filled out her Body Family Tree and her Body Timeline, and she reviewed a few Time Audits she'd filled out months before. She was relieved to see in black and white that she was the only one in her family who'd had breast cancer—so hers was less likely to be the most dangerous kind. She kicked herself a little when the Body Timeline pinpointed the exact moment she'd given up exercising: eight years beforehand, with the birth of her youngest by Caesarean section. Her daily walk ritual had been interrupted, and she'd never gotten it back on track.

But it was the Time Audit that gave her the most pause. For each of the three days she'd charted, there was not a *single hour* for herself. She saw very clearly that her entire life was absorbed by activities for other people. Laundry, cooking, shopping, cleaning. Soccer and swim practice. School library, PTA. Entertaining work guests, in-laws. Nowhere in any of those three days were the words, "Worked on art project" or "Researched courses" or even "Had dinner out with Rob." Lying alone in her bed, surgery wounds aching, Melissa started to cry. Somewhere along the way, she'd lost herself.

Melissa spent a sleepless night wondering what came next for her. She made a little deal with God: If you get me through this, I'm going to pull myself together.

When she woke up in the morning, she realized that she could use the Release program to help her recover from surgery. The timing was perfect, as the lighter meals worked well with her body's healing processes to help nudge her back into Positive Feedback. Instead of diverting energy to digest heavy meals, her system could send the nutrients from the program's health-supportive and anti-inflammatory foods straight to her wounds.

When she started feeling better, a process that was jump-started by an all-clear call from the doctor, Melissa resisted the temptation to jump out of bed and get right back into her demanding schedule. She forced herself to get more than eight hours of sleep a night, drank her lemon water, and did a modified Morning Glory routine, making sure not to get any water on her wounds, focusing instead on her meditations and visualizations. And she sat down to do Release the Time-Wasters on Your Time Audit and other Release exercises.

First, looking at all the pictures of happy children and the pieces of kid art she'd lovingly hung around the house, she forgave herself for "abandoning" her dreams for sixteen years—she had a pretty darn good excuse, after all—and started the process of letting go of any regrets about time she'd missed. She knew that this would be an ongoing process, but with her newfound gratitude—no cancer!—she was more excited than regretful. Then she set out a clear plan in her revised Time Audit: She was going to spend three hours this week researching the best school where she could finish her law degree.

When I saw her for the first time since her breast surgery—this was about two months later—she'd gotten a formal clean bill of health, and she'd already signed up to take the LSAT for entry into law school. She'd lost about ten pounds and had grown her hair out, gotten it straightened and colored—she looked ten years younger. While originally she'd considered a corporate law program, when Melissa did the Radiant Deep Dive (more on this later), she realized that her passion was immigration—she wanted to help people become American citizens. Her parents had come to the States in the 1960s and had struggled for years with understanding the system. She wanted to ensure that more low-income families like her own would have the chance to fulfill their dreams, just as she and her parents had.

"Vicky, I don't know how to describe it," she gushed. "I feel alive for the first time in a long, long while." Melissa had faced the worst of her pain, both emotionally and physically, and had come out the other side with a renewed understanding of her purpose, her passion. She loved her husband and her kids—but she was ready for more. And now she stood before me, absolutely radiant with excitement for her next phase.

When people get done with an in-person, hands-on treatment with me, using cupping, acupuncture, cranial sacral therapy, or some kind of deep tissue or spinal manipulation, many say something like, "Wow, Vicky—I feel alive. I feel like my whole body is glowing." They report later that friends told them, "It's like you're lit from within." And they *do* have a whole-body glow—their cheeks are rosier, their skin is smoother, their eyes are clearer, their hair is shinier. The Positive Feedback program taps into those same effects, and the results are just as visible. By the end of the program's three weeks, most people are getting the same kind of compliments. There's a difference, though: When you stimulate radiant effects, the results last longer and have the potential to change the course of your life.

Let's do a quick scan of where we are. You've been doing the Morning Glory ritual for two weeks, and it shows. You've released most of the toxins in your food. You've begun to let go of the stresses and distractions in your life and have started the work of refocusing on positive influences. As you've repeated this Release process over many days, you've gradually neutralized your body's stress response so that you feel less pain. Perhaps it's already become easier and more automatic to stay relaxed rather than get worried and anxious. While progressively toning the parasympathetic nervous system and the Adaptive Response, the Positive Feedback program has also been strengthening your resolve to maintain all the powerful, life-lengthening, beauty-enhancing changes in your eating, exercise, and overall wellness regimen.

As we've seen, the primary physical mechanism of Negative Feedback is inflammation. You've been doing everything you can to reverse inflammation and thus halt negativity's progression. Through the first two stages of the Positive Feedback program, you've put the brakes on the negative spiral, halting the inflammation that's causing your pain and giving your sympathetic nervous system a break. Your endocrine system has stopped churning out stress hormones that pad your belly and upper back with toxic fat. You're starting to experience the Positive Feedback cascade, and those endorphins and other mood-enhancing neuro-chemicals are restoring your body's healthiest settings.

Strengthening the parasympathetic system in this way not only allows you to release inflammation and anxiety—it also makes it easier for your brain to make good choices. Freed from the tyranny of the amygdala's hot temper, your brain's cool planning center, the prefrontal cortex, can help you do effective long-range planning. As you move into week 3: Radiate, your strengthened prefrontal cortex will help you summon even greater willpower to continue releasing harmful foods and toxic habits as well as help you cast your mind into the future, to see what comes next.

When you dive in and embrace the full scope of the Positive Feedback program and tap into your innate Adaptive Response, the results can be almost like a dream: The pounds fall off. Pain you've had for years resolves itself. You're ready to let go of traumas that you may have been carrying around for most of your life—and your body is ready and all too happy to let them go as well.

In the Radiate stage, you'll discover the strength and the clarity to live your life the way you've always hoped you could. You'll eat a diet composed entirely of anti-inflammatory foods, foods designed by nature to soothe inflamed tissues, foods so delicious you'll no longer be tempted by sugar or refined grains. Now that your Adaptive Response is once again fully engaged, and your diet is actively fighting inflammation, you can take your exercise to the next level, with a physical challenge that connects to your deeper purpose. This movement will rid you of any remaining accumulated pain and tension as well as help you firm your body and shed any excess pounds. You have done the work of letting go and preparing your body for an entirely new phase of strength!

Your entire body will soon radiate with health. You will look and feel the way you were born to be, the way you *deserve* to be.

The Radiate element is not only the culminating part of the Positive Feedback program, it's the active state that you will live in now that you've listened and responded to your pain. By radiating, you show the world who you are and what makes you alive and glorious. You become a bright and shining sun in your own world, radiating rays of powerful light all around you. That golden-white light that you welcome in during your meditation will now start to glow from within.

Let's see how you can help that inner beauty you've released radiate out to the world.

Finding Your Purpose

It's time to turn your focus outward. You've done a lot of introspection in the Reflect stage, and a lot of self-focused cleansing in Release. Now it's time to find your purpose and your passion, the driving force that will ground you and keep you happily in Positive Feedback for years to come.

Many of my patients say, "I have a job—*that's* my purpose." But is it? Are you truly satisfied and happy in your work, whether that's in your home or at a business? Or have you defaulted into a victim role, becoming a slave to your child or your boss? If you stay in that imbalanced place, it's only a matter of time before you slide back into the negative. Radiate work is about finding your anchor, your compass, the touchstone that will root you firmly in Positive Feedback no matter what life throws at you.

Discovering your purpose, your passion, your grounding is essential work—maybe even your primary task as a human being. Without this anchor, it's all too easy to lose yourself in your kids, partner, job, addictions—and slip back into the grip of your pain. So let's create a space for purpose that's constantly renewed with positive energy.

Positive Structure

As we did in the Release week, we'll begin Radiate structure work by adding an additional element to your Morning Glory ritual. My hope is that by this time in your program, that ritual is set in stone in your daily schedule. Have you begun to understand what I mean about Morning Glory being a foundation to your life? Does the ritual help you orient yourself toward self-care and the Reflect * Release * Radiate process every morning? It should feel like a daily reset, a way to get in touch with yourself and get grounded before you go out into the world.

ALTERNATING HOT AND COLD RINSES

Since you began the Morning Glory ritual in the Reflect week, you've been ending your daily shower with a cold-water rinse. Now I'd like you to be even more deliberate about the use of hot and cold. *Alternating* hot and cold water stimulates your blood vessels to expand and contract, boosting your circulation. The changing temperature, along with the pressure of the water, triggers the same effect in your lymphatic system, which has no pump and thus relies on this type of manual stimulation to keep things moving.

After you've completed your hair washing/conditioning and body wash, turn the water as hot as you can stand it, making sure to hit every part of your head and body. Then turn the cold as cold as it gets. (Don't worry: No matter how cold that water is, it can't hurt you.) Your lungs will expand to take in a deep breath to deal with the shock of the water, increasing your oxygen supply. The cold water will also stimulate the

Radiate-Week Morning Glory Ritual at a Glance

- Warm water with lemon
- Tibetan Rites
- Breathing exercise
- Daily reflection
- Dry brushing
- Shower
- Alternating hot and cold rinses
- Self-massage with oil
- Nine-point meditation

locus coeruleus, the so-called blue spot in the brain, an area known for releasing noradrenaline, a natural antidepressant. The noradrenaline released from the blue spot also suppresses neuroinflammation found in Alzheimer's,[1] and it's possible this mechanism may also be related to the glymphatic brain-cleansing system at work during sleep.[2]

Keep the cold on as long as you can; then switch it back to hot—again, as hot and as long as you can stand it. Do three to five full cycles of hot and cold water, each about thirty seconds long. Finish with a bracing, full-body cold drench. Studies have shown that regular cold-water bathing tones the sympathetic and parasympathetic nervous systems and stimulates the Adaptive Response, ultimately *decreasing* levels of stress hormones and inflammatory cytokines.[3] Cold water also stimulates the production of so-called brown fat cells, the "good" fat that increases our base metabolic rate, so we burn more calories all the time and stay leaner.

One patient of mine has his own version of this hydrotherapy: He takes a long run, then submerges his body in an ice bath, and then has a treatment with me. A bit extreme for me, but he swears by this practice!

TUMMY MASSAGE

The tummy massage is a controversial exercise among my patients. You absolutely must have your stomach massaged when you go for a treatment—otherwise you will not get the most from your lymphatic drainage. The gut needs to move. You wouldn't believe how many stunningly gorgeous women say, "Ugh! I don't want to touch my belly!" That attitude is exactly what this massage seeks to rectify. There should be *no* part of your body that makes you say, "Ugh," even your stomach. Assigning tummy massage is my way of forcing you to make friends with every part of your body—especially those parts that might have caused you some embarrassment in times past. Listen to me: *Every* part of you is beautiful. If you want to work on your stomach, that's another matter—but it still deserves your love.

Before you get dressed for the day, look in the mirror. Put your hands on your stomach and really *feel* your belly. Whether it's flat or full, firm or fleshy, apply your hands in a warm and loving way. Now, lie on the floor with knees bent. Give your belly just a loving little rub to warm it up. Start from the right lower side, next to the right ovary, between the hip bone and pubic bone. Put fingers close together, almost in a cup, and press gently, making little circular clockwise movements. Move your fingers slightly up, and repeat over and over as you move from your lower right up to the top of your rib cage, across to your diaphragm, over to your left side, and then down. Continue in this patter, making a shape like a snail on your belly, until you finish by your belly button.

Positive Function

As in the earlier weeks of the program, the Radiate week addresses positive function primarily through those things that we take into our body. Changes in intake that might seem small to one person can be direly threatening to another.

One week, I had three women with the exact same pain profile: They all suffered with bladder and urinary tract infections, and they all had constipation. Furthermore, they were all anemic, were kind of pale, and had lower back pain. And all had a tendency to love their red wine.

These three women had different stories and situations, but they all had issues with trust and lack of forgiveness toward their mothers (who in each case had abandoned them emotionally in some fundamental way). Their lives were ruled by fear: Fear of being abandoned. Fear of letting go. Fear of losing control. They were all very stubborn, stuck in their ways—and all craved alcohol and the wrong foods.

Perhaps you've guessed this by now, but the hardest thing for all three was not releasing their pain—it was changing their diet. ("It's the only pleasure I have left!")

The work I do with my patients who are addicted to inflammatory foods often follows a specific pattern: They balk at the Release program but, after I give them a pep talk and remind them of the effects of poor dietary choices, leave my office determined to make it happen. In a week or two, they're back with big smiles, bristling with energy, their tummies less bloated, their skin and hair shining brighter than in years. They've finally made the connection: You are what you eat. I've seen it happen again and again and again. Once you start avoiding all inflammatory foods, your body will enjoy and even crave the taste of healthy foods. You have begun to *radiate*.

We choose the foods we eat based on one of three reasons: health, pleasure, or spirituality.[4] In a way, the Radiate component of the Positive Feedback program brings all three of these factors together into an eating program that makes your taste buds, your body, and even your soul radiate. When we remember to eat mindfully and savor every bite mindfully (or at least the first few bites), we intensify the pleasure of the food, and our lives become more radiant, too.

Now that you've completed the Release Meal Plan, your body has likely moved out of the inflammatory state brought on by toxic foods. You can now move into the Radiate Meal Plan (the second half of chapter 7). You'll notice that there are many, many options and varieties in the menus and food lists. That's because this approach to eating will be with you for the rest of your life.

One major difference between the Release and the Radiate plans is the inclusion of more lean protein in the latter, especially foods rich in omega-3s. The Radiate Meal Plan is based largely upon the Mediterranean style of eating. (Of course! I am Greek, after all.) With a focus on fresh vegetables and fruits, lean meats (especially omega-3-rich fish), whole grains, and monounsaturated fats (such as olive oil), and avoidance of refined grains and sugars, the Mediterranean approach to eating is the most balanced, anti-pain, anti-inflammatory approach you can find. (And scores of studies have proven it!)

I love the gorgeous foods included in this approach—especially fruits such as pineapple, blueberries, raspberries. I love eating brown rice, with its nourishing and nutty nature. I love my walnuts, my almonds, my figs. I love goji berries. I don't feel like it's a *diet* thing; I feel like it's happy food. I love these foods, not only because they're incredibly delicious, but because they love my body back.

The only variation from the standard Mediterranean fare in my approach is that I do *not* advocate cow's-milk dairy, nor do I include wheat, barley, and rye as acceptable grains, because of reactivity to dairy proteins and to gluten. The anti-gluten focus is still slightly controversial: Some experts believe that the only people who have problems with wheat are those with celiac disease (an autoimmune condition that causes severe reactivity to gluten) or with true gluten intolerance (which is itself a bit controversial). But I've seen the difference among my patients. Foods with gluten tend to cause bloating and puffiness. As soon as a patient releases gluten from her diet, the features of her face come back into focus, the redness in her skin and nose fades a bit, and her eyes are clearer and less obscured by pillowy eyelids.

The nearby tables give a range of selected Positive Feedback proteins (table 7), complex carbohydrates (table 8), and vegetables and fruits (table 9); these are the sorts of foods you'll be consuming on the Positive Feedback Meal Plan outlined in chapter 7. If you're feeling confident that you have a good handle on the principles of the Positive Feedback Meal Plan (which, as noted earlier, appears in both a Release and a Radiate version in the next chapter), and you're yearning to experiment with additional foods, flip through the recipe section for inspiration (chapter 8). Alternatively, if you've moved beyond following a prescribed meal plan and are eager to transition to designing your own meals, use the food lists in tables 7 through 9 to help you select your favorite foods.

In general, try not to get "stuck" on any one food. A diverse diet is your best food ally. If you eat too much of any one food, you can develop a reactivity to it. Try to rotate foods as often as is practical and affordable for you. For example, alternate your snacks—one day walnuts, the next day pecans, then cashews, then walnuts, and so on.

Table 7. **Positive Feedback Proteins**

POSITIVE FEEDBACK PROTEINS	SOURCES	BENEFITS
Eggs	Organic free-range (four per week)	Rich in lutein (yolks) for brain health; high in omega-3s (with free-range having ten times as much as non-free-range)
Goat's-milk (and related products)	Goat's-milk feta and mozzarella (avoid all other dairy products with the exception of live yogurt, below)	High prevalence of beneficial bacteria; good source of protein for vegetarians; good dopamine trigger (for focus and motivation)
Lean meat	100 percent grass-fed beef, buffalo, goat, venison (twice per week)	Lower in fat and calories than grain-fed, with additional antioxidants and omega-3s; higher in fat-burning conjugated linoleic acids and iron
Lean poultry	Organic turkey (once or twice per week) and chicken (once per week)	High in protein, low in calories; free of bacterial infestations that plague nonorganic poultry as a result of overcrowding and overuse of antibiotics
Live yogurt	Organic sheep's- or goat's-milk yogurt containing no more than 2 percent fat	Packed with probiotics to strengthen the immune system and combat leaky gut
Nuts and seeds	Almonds, cashews, Brazil nuts, walnuts, hazelnuts, pine nuts, pistachios, macadamia nuts, sunflower seeds, pumpkin seeds, sesame seeds, flaxseed, chia seeds, pecans	Rich in good fiber and omega-3s; helpful in reducing inflammation
Oily fish	Tuna, sardines, mackerel, salmon, whitefish, monkfish, cod, red snapper (twice per week total)	Rich in omega-3s and polyunsaturated fats that reduce inflammation and improve cardiac and neurologic health

(continued)

Table 7. **Positive Feedback Proteins** (*continued*)

POSITIVE FEEDBACK PROTEINS	SOURCES	BENEFITS
Vegetable sources	Black-eyed peas, adzuki beans, green beans, broccoli, spinach, kale, other leafy greens	Helpful in lowering blood sugar and decreasing oxidative stress by lowering cytokines
Complete-protein combinations	Beans and cheese; brown rice and seeds; brown rice and beans; quinoa dishes; cheese, nuts, and seeds and a variety of mixed vegetables	Capable of meeting your protein needs without meat

Table 8. **Positive Feedback Complex Carbohydrates**

POSITIVE FEEDBACK COMPLEX CARBOHYDRATES	SOURCES	BENEFITS
Bread	Spelt bread, yeast-free rye bread, whole-grain flourless breads	Low in gluten content
Grains	Oats, pearl spelt	Helpful in lowering blood sugar; packed with hard-to-find soluble fiber
Pasta	Millet and spelt pasta, soba noodles (100 percent buckwheat)	Enable pasta without the guilt!
Rice	Organic brown, basmati, and wild rice	Contain more fiber and nutrients than white rice

Table 9. **Positive Feedback Vegetables and Fruits**

POSITIVE FEEDBACK VEGETABLES AND FRUITS	SOURCES	BENEFITS
Green	Spinach, Swiss chard, green beans, broccoli, kale, collard greens, turnip greens, romaine, cabbage, amaranth, celery, bok choy, Brussels sprouts, quinoa, radicchio, endive, arugula, fennel, grapes, kiwis, apples, avocados, artichokes, broccoli rabe, cucumbers, pears, limes, asparagus, zucchini	Rich in lutein, potassium, vitamins C and K, and folic acid
Orange/Yellow	Sweet potatoes, tangerines, peaches, winter squash, carrots, cantaloupe, pineapple, pumpkin, papaya, star fruit, mangoes	Rich in beta-carotene and vitamin C; support immune system, vision
Purple/Blue	Red cabbage, purple kale, purple carrots, "blue" corn, grapes, blueberries	High in anti-aging, anti-cancer phytochemicals; support mental clarity
Red	Pomegranate, grapefruit, tomato, peppers, beets, red onions, radishes, rhubarb, watermelon, strawberries, raspberries, cherries, lingonberries, figs, goji berries	Source of potent antioxidants: lycopene and anthocyanins
White	White asparagus, garlic, cauliflower, turnips, onions, parsnips, and kohlrabi	Rich in phytochemicals and potassium; reduce cholesterol, lower blood pressure, and prevent diabetes

REINTRODUCING REACTIVE FOODS

After the Release stage and at the start of your Radiate work is actually the best time to test for reactivity. Pull out your Food Diary from the Reflect week and note again the foods on your list that corresponded with negative moods (lethargy, anger, irritation, weepiness) or negative physical symptoms (swelling in fingers or feet, painful muscles or joints, receding gums, headaches, lower back pain, excess gas/stomach upset, sleep disturbance). Based on how you reacted when you ate these foods the first time, are you certain you want to reintroduce them? For example, I've realized that I'm reactive to cruciferous vegetables, so cauliflower, Brussels sprouts, and cabbage are permanently off the menu for me. Continue to listen to your body after eating. Note—and eliminate—those foods that make you feel bad.

If reaction-causing foods are among your favorites, you might nonetheless consider making a clean break now—you have the opportunity (and may have the willpower, given your current focus on healthy eating) to simply wipe them out of your life. If you want to be absolutely certain that a beloved food is at fault, try this method:

Day 1: Eat a single serving of the food in question. Take careful notes of mood, physical symptoms, appetite, etc.

Day 2: Without eating any more of the food in question, take careful notes of mood, physical symptoms, appetite, etc.

Day 3: Take careful notes of mood, physical symptoms, appetite, etc.

Day 4: Try another serving of the food. Take careful notes of mood, physical symptoms, appetite, etc.

Study these new notes. If you find many of the same descriptors on all four days, as well as many days in the original Food Diary listings—in other words, no change—chances are that your beloved food is *not* the reactivity culprit. However, if you've noted changes in your body and state of mind within twelve hours of eating a specific food, and those same

Can't Find Organic Almond Milk? Make Your Own!

One of the frustrating parts about being an almond milk lover is seeing how some companies can take something so healthy and turn it bad by adding tons of sugar. I am lucky to have access to fresh unsweetened almond milk, but if you don't, try this at home:

Buy 2 to 3 pounds of raw organic almonds. (Always buy organic—the flavor is better, and you don't have to worry about the chemicals!) Soak the almonds overnight in filtered water, filling the bowl until the water is about 2 inches higher than the almonds. Soaking releases the enzymes, so it is a very important step. In the morning, pour the entire mixture (almonds and water) into a food processor or strong blender (like a Vitamix, the ultimate health tool!). Begin slow, making sure the top of the blender is secure. Turn up to high slowly, then leave on for about 2 to 3 minutes. (When you are done, scoop out the top foam for the best cappuccino of your life!)

Take a glass Ball jar (or similar) and put a tea strainer over the top. (You can also use a cheesecloth, but I like the ritual and simplicity of the strainer.) Pour the mixture in slowly, and keep turning around the mush with a spoon—the milk will drop into the glass jar. Sometimes I add water to the soaked almonds to get the right consistency. Just keep doing the straining until you have about 32 ounces—enough for 2 days! (Once it's completed, I don't keep more than 2 days.)

This wonder elixir is way more than a milk. I use almond milk in soups, tea, and just drink a small glass to balance my blood sugar if I am ever tempted by the wrong foods. You might add a little organic vanilla extract or cinnamon for added sweetness. Pour it into your green smoothies for a creamy texture and a nice change.

Almonds rock!

The Positive Feedback To-Go Plan

If you feel that you don't have time to do the entire plan—not yet anyway—keep these ten points in mind and you won't fall any further into Negative Feedback.

1. Increase intake of fluids to eight to ten glasses a day.

2. Improve sleep by changing an uncomfortable mattress or pillow and increasing ventilation in your bedroom (opening a bedroom or bathroom window to allow fresh air to circulate).

3. Take a power nap. Steal time for yourself by setting aside thirty minutes each day for breathing/meditation.

4. Take regular walks and avoid sitting in one position for too long.

5. For any injuries or pain, think of the acronym RICE: rest, ice, compression, elevate. Apply an ice pack for twenty minutes three times a day to the injury; avoid applying ice directly to the skin. Wrap a sprain or a twist with an Ace bandage, or wear compression stockings, to contain inflammation.

6. Relax by taking a hot bath with lavender and Epsom salts two or three evenings a week.

7. Increase protein intake by eating organic red meats such as turkey (not smoked), grass-fed beef, lamb, or veal a few times a week.

8. Lower your carbohydrate intake by switching to brown rice and/or quinoa with meals.

9. Increase egg-white omelet consumption and include goat's-milk cheese in your diet on a weekly basis.

10. Have health-promoting snacks available at the office, including baby figs, walnuts, almonds, goji berries, blueberries, raspberries, and goat's-milk yogurt. A spoonful of honey and a sprinkle of cinnamon may be added if wished. (Snacks should be taken at approximately 11:00 A.M. and 3:30 P.M. daily.)

changes are found in the corresponding spot in your Food Diary, *and* they duplicate themselves on the fourth day of your test sequence, I'm afraid you have a reactivity. To be sure, eliminate the food in question for three weeks. Then, introduce it for two days, carefully noting your symptoms. Then eliminate it again and see if you feel any different. The answer should be very clear.

If you are still not sure, consider exploring a food sensitivity blood test, done by a lab. These tests are not covered by insurance and are still very controversial; many have conflicting findings. Talk to your doctor or allergist for more information. (They are likely to advise a food elimination test!)

Again, just as with pain, try to see this as a helpful outcome that's yielding priceless information. Remember what happened to me when I ignored my physical symptoms from Granny's cakes and pies: I suffered with eczema and bloatedness . Your body will allow itself to be ignored for just so long. Better to know now than when you have to go under for surgery.

Now that your diet is running on all cylinders, I'm eager for you to stretch yourself a bit and reach for a new physical challenge that connects with you on a deeper level. Let's move on to the motion component of your Radiate week.

Positive Motion

You've spent two weeks taking it easy (exertion-wise)—doing the Tibetan Rites, going for short walks, and/or doing gentle yoga—in order to let your sympathetic nervous system relax and your inflammation ratchet down a few notches. Hopefully by now you can feel a difference in your body—perhaps a bit less pain? Are your joints feeling stronger? Do you notice any differences when you get out of bed?

If your pains *are* decreasing and you *are* feeling more energetic from the Positive Feedback changes you've made, it's time to consider what's next for you physically. Remember, the basic tenet of Adaptive Response is *challenge,* so you need to be pushing yourself a bit more all the time to continue to derive the biggest benefit.

For some of you, challenge may take the form of an extra three cycles of Tibetan Rites; for others, perhaps you'll extend your morning walk to thirty minutes or shoot for 10,000 steps a day. But for others of you—particularly the women who've missed their sweaty workouts—once you've reached your twenty-one repetitions of the Tibetan Rites, start thinking about other ways you can move your body through space in a way that will also send your soul aloft.

If you're a runner, how long has it been since you did a run for charity—and really gave your all to the fundraising effort? Perhaps you've done a 5K here and there but haven't really paid attention to the cause. Or perhaps you've done lots of smaller races, but what you've really wanted to try was a triathlon. For any particular disorder or disability, you can find a run, walk, or other kind of race organized for fundraising. One I find particularly inspiring is Team in Training, from the Leukemia and Lymphoma Society. If you sign up for one of their races, you have access to a wonderful mentor program, with coaches, training regimens, workout partners, and other varied supports—but the organization requires you to raise several thousand dollars to participate. The investment of physical and mental time makes this endeavor all-consuming—and life-changing.

Or perhaps you like to take the occasional walk in the woods. How about trying a multiday backpacking trip? You could chart out a couple days on the Appalachian Trail or the Pacific Crest Trail and cover considerable ground using just your own two feet. Or gather a group of women to go to Machu Picchu and climb on the ruins. Anything that speaks to your soul and challenges your body is an appropriate task for motion work in the Radiate stage. The goal is to pick an activity that will help you do the following:

Work toward a physical goal: Setting a physical target several months in advance will make it easier for you to stick with the

Positive Feedback program. The longer you can maintain new habits, the more likely they are to stick.

Look forward to a future, extraordinary event: Research has found that anticipation of a future fun event often brings us more happiness than the event itself![5]

Transfer that accomplishment to other big goals: Working toward something that's just outside your comfort zone will help the Adaptive Response strengthen not just your body, but also your *will*. You'll see that you're capable of so much—you just need to believe in yourself.

Bring your mind into your body: You gain a feeling of wholeness and integration when you're working toward a goal you love with your heart and your head.

Whatever activity you choose, I hope that you experience an endorphin rush again, and fall in love with it. You knew that rush as a child, and you likely experienced it often as a young adult. You deserve to feel it again. That rush comes not only from pushing yourself physically, but also from achieving a goal that two weeks earlier might not have seemed possible.

Positive Emotion

Now, in the Radiate stage, is your time to shine. I'd love for you to make it a habit to radiate positive emotion and become an expressive outlet for your life story. What's your passion? What's your story? How will you tell it to everyone you meet?

One of the most vivid memories I have from childhood is seeing Mom in a yoga handstand for several minutes every day. I used to marvel at her strength and focus. When I was about six years old, my favorite game was to dress up (simultaneously) as a nurse and a flight attendant. I'd gather up my toy suitcase and one of my dolls and proclaim, "I'm a nurse today, and I'm traveling to America to heal this patient." I love this memory because in many ways I've taken the best of both parents' life work—Dad traveling, coaching people on how to use their bodies; Mom sharing all she knew about nutrition, meditation, and yoga—and I've combined those facets into a practice that allows me to help people all over the world.

Ever since I was a child, I've gravitated toward people who were equally passionate about their work. I love dropping my boys off at school so that I can get a chance to talk briefly with their teachers. Teachers are such inspiring people: Their main purpose, their whole job, is to employ different techniques to bring the best out of people. When teachers love what they do, it's their passion, their gift—and that passion helps them do even better by their students.

The core of teaching is helping others, and I really believe that that's the most radiant work we can do. When you love something as much as most helping professionals love their work, you don't do it for the money. You want to share your positive intention and good energy with everybody around you. When you're doing radiant work, you don't wake up and go to work and say, "Oh God, I've got to teach these twenty-five kids today, *again*." When you do radiant work, you do it with passion and love.

So the primary work of the emotion component of the Radiate stage is answering the question, "What is that thing bigger than yourself that you can (and want to) pour your heart and soul into?" Ultimately, I'd like you to be able to say this meditation to yourself:

I do wonderful work in a wonderful way for which I receive wonderful pay.

RADIANT DEEP DIVE

One of my patients, a thirty-five-year-old woman named Zoe, had gone down the negative path of not feeling appreciated by husband and kids. She was casting about for something to make her feel alive again—and that something looked very much like an affair.

She'd just had a baby within the past year, and somewhere, deep down, I believe she was afraid she was losing her beauty. She talked to me about a guy she knew from the neighborhood, about wanting to find a lover so that she could lose herself and feel sexy again. Zoe thought her husband didn't want her anymore; he was content with her being the mother of his kids, nothing more.

Thankfully, we had this discussion before she acted on her thoughts and actually started an affair. As we talked, she thought about how an affair would devastate her family, and she realized that she herself would only get hurt and emotionally involved, which would lead to tears and pain. So she decided to go back to what *really* was missing in her life, which was her passion: being a buyer for a department store. She realized that her passion, her job, her office, her team were where she felt safe and grounded. She loved being a mom, but she also loved being an independent woman who had her own time to go to the gym, her own money, and no one to tell her what to do. Doing her Radiant Deep Dive, she realized that she'd fallen into the trap of being lonely at home. Made aware of her feelings through our discussions, she realized what had happened in time to channel this drive in a positive way, instead of in a way that might have destroyed her marriage.

To do your Deep Dive, take out your Time Audit—both your original and your revised versions. And then sit down, close your eyes, and think of the happiest day of your life *as a child*. Try to recreate it mentally in as much detail as possible to answer these questions:

1. Where are you?

2. Who is with you?

3. What time of day is it? Time of year?

4. What are you wearing?

5. What are you doing?

6. Are you excited because of what you're doing, or who you're with, or for some other reason?

7. If you could do this activity right now, where would you be?

8. Who would you be with?

9. If money were no object, where would you be standing right now?

10. What would you have done today if you didn't have to conduct your ordinary routine?

11. Where would you be going tomorrow?

Open your eyes and just sit for a moment; be still. Take a deep breath, all the way in and out. Now look at your revised Time Audit, the one you created with the activities in your ideal day. Do the activities on this sheet reflect the vision you just summoned in your head? How can you merge your childhood best day with your current best day? What would it take to get there?

I do this Deep Dive with my patients because even when people talk about how they'd like to spend their days as adults, they don't tend to give credence to childhood dreams—when, in fact, that's where our deepest passions lie waiting for us. Spend some time developing that Time Audit for your childhood best day, and you just may discover your true passion.

BRAINSTORMING YOUR RADIANT LIFE

Sometimes when people get done with these exercises, they're still not quite sure what should come next. Maybe you've completed the first two phases—reflected on your past and released your emotional pain—but you're still asking yourself, What now? Where do I go from here?

These huge questions can take you a lifetime to answer, but there's help: Researchers are looking into how we humans can create satisfying lives for ourselves. Dr. Martin Seligman, author of *Learned Optimism and Authentic Happiness,* is a professor at the University of Pennsylvania and a pioneer in the field of positive psychology.[6] Positive psychology encourages us to zero in on and expand the things that give us joy and contentment, rather than trying to eradicate the things that hurt us. In his work, he has identified three ways through which we can develop our path to happiness:

- The pleasant life, in which we sink deeply into, amplify, and intensify our pleasures—the path chosen by, say, a "foodie"

- The engaged life, in which we sink deeply into "flow" experiences—the path of a musician, an artist, or a gardener

- The meaningful life, in which we sink deeply into our service to others, seeking to dedicate ourselves to a larger cause—the path of a community organizer, a philanthropist, or even a hands-on mom or dad

When we focus our lives around a *combination* of these three factors, we tend to experience greater, more long-lasting satisfaction. This research can really help you zero in on what makes you come alive. What's your purpose? Why are you here? What gives you pleasure? What allows you to lose yourself in the moment? What makes you shine?

If you need still more prompts, ask yourself: What do I love about myself? To get at the heart of this, try writing a letter to your future self: What do you want your children or grandchildren to be able to say about you?

Ask yourself, What is it that I can do all day long and time seems to stand still? Is it art, music, writing, dance, drama, gardening, cooking, sports? Do I love to be with children or elderly people? Do I love collaborating on big projects? Do I like spending time alone, working on a puzzle that I alone can solve?

Once you pin down that passion, ask yourself, How can I do more of that? How can I share the gift of that passion with the world?

If you find it difficult to see the path from where you are now to where you want to be, do what teachers do with their kids: Break it down into baby steps.

BABY STEPS

Stating a goal is the first step toward making something happen.

In your notebook, start with the biggest possible articulation of the goal.

- I want to become an astronaut.

Then keep breaking it down into smaller goals:

- I want to become an astrophysicist.

- I want to get a graduate degree.

- I want to get accepted to graduate school.

- I want to finish college.

Once you've walked the goal all the way back to where you are now (let's say, studying for finals on your last college course), make a list of the five smallest things you can do to make that next goal happen. (Sharpen pencils for test; finish studying for test; take test; hand in test; order graduation gown.)

Once you've enjoyed your graduation party, cross finishing college off the list and move up one level. Break down that *next* goal into smaller steps. Then, systematically, keep taking those small steps, goal by goal, rewriting your lists in your notebook often so that you can rechart your course as necessary.

Do those baby steps sound too small? The researchers at Stanford's Persuasive Tech Lab have been studying behavior change, and they've found that the way to make positive, lasting changes is to break those changes into microscopic units and then repeat those mini-steps until they have a place in your daily life.[7] For example, if you want to commit to flossing your teeth, floss one tooth—just one. Then, tomorrow, floss that one tooth again. And again. Every time you complete the tiny task, you get a little shot of dopamine in your brain (that hormone linked to pleasure, ambition, and addiction). Yep—you're creating your own little addiction to success with every achieved tiny goal.

Eventually, you'll have a habit, and you'll be flossing up a storm. (*And you'll be on your way to the moon!*)

Now that you've created the vision, and broken down the steps, there's only one thing missing: for you to share it with someone you love.

INVESTING IN RADIANT RELATIONSHIPS

My mom helped me develop a strong "contentment system," the term I shared in chapter 1 that Paul Gilbert uses to describe a well-toned nervous system. When your contentment system is strong, it allows you to feel safe and soothed every day. Your orientation is on finding and maintaining strong, nurturing connections. Thanks to the work of my mom, my entire being was calibrated and preset to exist in Positive Feedback. Ever since I left home, I've spent my life trying to share this blessing with others.

In contrast, many of my patients were raised in households that favored the "drive system"—focused on achieving goals and increasing resources. This type of orientation can be exciting and motivating, but can wear you down if you press the accelerator for too long. Or, worse, they were raised in homes leaning toward the "threat system"—characterized by anxiety, anger, and disgust, focused primarily on threats. When your threat system predominates, you grow up feeling on edge, jumpy, and suspicious, focusing all your energy on finding safety—and you can be pre-programmed for Negative Feedback.

When I'm working with my patients, thirty years later, I rely upon the strength I got from my mom—from her genes, but also from her very contentment-system-focused parenting, all of the meditation and positive affirmations, all the nutritious, anti-inflammatory foods, and focus on exercise and relaxation. But while you may have grown up with parents who were either focused on the drive system or, sadly, the threat system, by now you hopefully recognize that everyone can go back and do it over again. You can all re-parent yourself and strengthen your contentment system with the Positive Feedback plan. I hope you're basking in the glow of a strengthened contentment system right now, and you recognize how much sweeter, softer, and safe life can feel in Positive Feedback. Strengthening your personal connections with others will help you sustain those changes for a lifetime.

We spend so much time and energy being nice to other people at work that we sometimes forget to be nice to the people closest to us! My mom and my grandma are the two women who've inspired me most in my life; they found what they liked to do early on, and they found a way to share that passion with other people. They would always say, *"Give to people and love people"* (especially my mom—such a love bug!). I've seen my mom take great care of all our aging relatives—her aunts and her mother, other elders in our town. My granny did the same. Their compassion and dedication transferred over to me, and I can feel that same sense of dedication and purpose when I treat my own clients.

I love my job, and I credit my good situation to the fact that I visualized where I wanted to be and who I wanted to be working with. You might say that I brought these beautiful people into my life. I believe that positive energy attracts positive energy, and that God sends us the right people at the right time.

That is the core of radiant living: Your light shines out into the world as you go about your work and follow your dreams. Your passion and energy attract your soul mates, your best friends, your most compatible colleagues and collaborators. You surround yourself with strong and soulful people, and you all, together, support one another in your Positive Feedback way of life. That contentment system of amazing power continues to strengthen and push you ever higher toward your goals.

Check-In: Are You Ready to Live in Positive Feedback—for Life?

I hope that you're feeling strong and ready to embrace the next phase of your life with passion and purpose. I can't tell you how rewarding it is for me to see or hear about someone moving all the way through the Reflect * Release * Radiate process and coming out the other end with an entirely new life. To inspire you, let me leave you with a story of one of my most inspiring patients, a woman I'll call Lisa. Lisa has moved all the way through the Positive Feedback sequence, and she's currently building a radiant life with a new body and a new love. But not too long ago, she was in dire physical and emotional straits. She'd been living in Negative Feedback for most of her life.

When she first came to me, Lisa told me she felt very dizzy. She would be out and about and would lose her balance, and then she'd start to feel nauseated, occasionally even vomiting. She'd been seeing someone for her panic, but her condition didn't seem to be improving at all. She had also been suffering with her neck pain and thyroid issues, and now she had fractured the big toe of her right foot, a trigger point for the liver. All her symptoms were classic signs of those irritability and aggressive tendencies that I call an "angry liver."

Lisa had started drinking white wine rather routinely, perhaps (she thought) more than she should. She felt unable to make decisions. She was dating a man who wasn't respecting her. She had hit a point where the pain in her body was screaming at her.

I sat her down with all the practitioners in our clinic and talked through her issues. We wanted to make sure we had the whole picture of Lisa's life and why she was in pain. I drew a diagram of Lisa's Body Timeline on a whiteboard. As we talked, it became clear that Lisa had never told her GP the most formative experience of her life: When Lisa was fourteen, she'd watched her best friend die in a car accident.

Her parents were away traveling at the time. Lisa was very upset, and asked her parents to come home and be with her. They didn't, and she was devastated—and then she was furious. She decided to send herself to boarding school—whether to punish her family or herself, I'm not sure. Without missing a beat, she continued on to college, then graduate school. She became a titan of business, but she'd rarely had contact with her family since the accident. She had developed a tough shell around an incredibly fragile core.

After many years of workaholism and pushing herself to the brink, Lisa had finally gone to the doctor. Experiencing severe burnout, she had been so exhausted that she couldn't get out of bed. Her GP referred her to an endocrinologist. After several months of treatment, that specialist had balanced Lisa's hormones, but she was now on antidepressants. And *still* she couldn't get out of bed.

Lisa was suffering. She was a managing director at her company at only thirty-four, with a whole division reporting to her. Her boyfriend was cold and removed, making her feel insecure and unloved. Her body was reacting to the rigorous demands she placed on it, which all started with her emotional issues. She needed to start loving herself and her parents more. She needed to release her draining relationship. She needed to face the trauma and anger of her past so that she could move on emotionally. As she was worked through her pain, I encouraged her to feel every bit of the anger—and boy, did she.

Once we made her Body Timeline, we had the information that we needed to talk about how Lisa could move forward. Using test results contributed by her GP, we realized that Lisa had thyroid issues, which an ultrasound confirmed.

Soon after our group consultation, Lisa set about serious Release work: She began processing the trauma of witnessing her friend's death with a therapist trained in eye motion desensitization and reprocessing (EMDR), a modality introduced in chapter 5 that helps to release trapped memories. The fact that she'd witnessed that horrific accident was life-changing—as was the fact that she'd wanted her parents to come home and help her heal from that event and they refused. Both of those experiences were equally traumatic, and equally trapped within her body tissues. And now Lisa was finally, after twenty years, getting help with all of it.

Lisa did the Reflect work and discovered the lessons of her pain. She was able to release the pain and forgive her parents (and herself). She gave her unloving boyfriend the boot. And once we cleaned up her diet and all the medication she was on, we started to talk about how to move into the future:

Instead of taking medication, she started drinking smoothies and taking vitamin D and fish oil (carefully following her GP's advice as she made the transition).

Instead of drinking Diet Coke, she relished nettle tea.

Instead of eating at her desk and working until seven or eight every night, she started making dinner plans with friends at delicious vegetarian restaurants, where nourishing foods were plentiful and white bread was rare, so she didn't have to say no to her beloved baguettes.

Once she started taking these steps, radiance was right there to greet her. She did her Radiant Deep Dive and realized that what she wanted more than anything was a family. She created a meditation to help her visualize her new reality:

Open my way. Let love and happiness come my way. Let me marry, have children and a man to love and to adore me. When the time is right, when I am ready, please, send him to me. Thank you, God.

The universe provided (as it tends to when we're receptive), and now—a year later—she and her high school sweetheart are married and planning to get pregnant. She's preparing her body for a healthy pregnancy by following the Positive Feedback program. She knows that reducing inflammation, releasing toxins from her body and brain, and resetting her parasympathetic nervous system before she gets pregnant could make a big difference in her baby's lifelong health.

Before she gets pregnant, as she prepares her body, Lisa is enjoying her radiance to the fullest. She's training for a 5K—by running barefoot! And after hiding for years in drab clothes of black and navy, she hired a stylist to add color to her wardrobe. She feels safe with her new man, who exudes a love and respect for her that her previous boyfriend never did.

A year ago, Lisa was still struggling in the dark, but she says now it seems obvious: She had to be willing to really *feel* the pain, to hit rock bottom and release those old wounds, in order to find herself. And that's exactly what she did. Lisa knows that as long as she follows her program, does her Morning Glory ritual, and sticks to her Radiate food lists, she'll remain in Positive Feedback. And now, so will her baby—and thus begins a whole new generation of contented, connected radiant health.

So simple, and so powerful. So life-changing.

So what's *your* story?

You've made it through a very challenging program, and a new world has opened up to you. The same structure of the Positive Feedback program that made it safe for you to wade through the truth of your pain will provide security to you as you boldly go forward and take risks in your new future.

You have a framework for an eating plan that will not only help you release pain and avoid disease, but also give you enough energy and vitality to fuel your newfound passions. You have a sustainable, progressive plan for your fitness; no matter how much you challenge yourself physically, the plan will help your body be there to meet you, step by step.

Living in the positive means that you know what works for you. You believe in yourself. You've found your positive voice—that calm, strong, optimistic feeling deep inside.

You feel free, safe, and grounded. At any time, if you encounter a problem that feels too large, or a pain that feels too raw, you can retrace your path through the Positive Feedback program and get a foothold again.

You know that every new day brings a new chance to restore yourself with the Morning Glory ritual.

You now have space in your body; you have a structure, a routine. You like being alone so that you can meditate, pray; you love being with others to feel connected and loved. You like starting your day with dry brushing and Tibetan rites, with foods that make you happy. Even the scale is happy. And if you have your once-a-week chocolate croissant, the voice of positivity says, "Don't worry; go back to your routine and everything will work its way back."

The path back to yourself can always start, and start again, with that first glass of warm water with lemon. Armed with all the work you've done in these three weeks, you won't find yourself back where you started even if you have a relapse. You've come too far to turn back. Nothing can stop you now. You're ready to share your radiance with the world.

Positivity always works. Your blood is flowing; your heart is beating. You are alive and happy; everything works.

Please look at yourself in the mirror and say this one last meditation with me:

I am confident. I am happy. I am ready to go.
I am the power and the authority in my life!

I believe in you. But, more important,
you believe in yourself.

PART THREE

The Positive Feedback Tools

7

The Positive Feedback Meal Plan

T he foods you consume have a significant impact on your body's ability to heal itself. If you're suffering from muscle and/or joint pain, food can help—*if* you choose wisely. That's where the Positive Feedback Meal Plan comes in. It will help you stop feeding your emotions acidic foods such as oranges, vinegar, alcohol, coffee, and colas, and junk foods that are high in sugar and wheat. All these foods, which exacerbate the inflammation causing your pain, are replaced by healthier options in the Positive Feedback Meal Plan. As we've discussed throughout the book, Positive Feedback eating is powered almost exclusively by anti-inflammatory foods.

My Mum's Voice: Raise Your Glass

Go ahead and pour yourself a glass of champagne or wine—and enjoy it. Remember, however, what the ancient Greeks used to say: "The first glass is for health, the second for love, the third for sleep, and the fourth for swearing."

This chapter contains two versions of the Positive Feedback Meal Plan. The first is for use during your Release week (though the meals from this version can be used at any time); the second is for the Radiate week and beyond.

The Release Meal Plan

As you will recall, in the first week of the Positive Feedback program—the Reflect week—you made no major dietary changes; instead, you reflected on your customary eating habits. Now, in the Release week, you

Table 10. **The Release Meal Plan**

DAY	UPON WAKING	AFTER WALKING	BREAKFAST
Monday	Liver Flush Smoothie	Tea of your choice (see options in table 17)	Either *no* breakfast (to increase the cleansing action), or ½ cup millet or oatmeal eaten an hour later than usual
Tuesday	Liver Flush Smoothie	Tea	Either *no* breakfast (to increase the cleansing action), or ½ cup millet or oatmeal eaten an hour later than usual
Wednesday	Liver Flush Smoothie	Tea	Either *no* breakfast (to increase the cleansing action), or ½ cup millet or oatmeal eaten an hour later than usual
Thursday through Sunday	Warm water with juice of ½ lemon	Tea	Smoothie of your choice (recipes in table 12)

will be eating a more modest number of foods, in order to enhance the cleansing action of the program. The Release Meal Plan is outlined in table 10.

Fair warning: The first three days, also known as the Liver Flush, sometimes trigger a few extra toilet visits! Bear that in mind when planning your outings. I would also recommend keeping your restaurant visits to a minimum during those days so that you can better control your access to Liver Flush foods.

For the remainder of the first week, I encourage you to experiment with a variety of smoothies (see recipes in table 12, later in this chapter) and get comfortable with your knife set—you're going to be doing a lot of

LUNCH	SNACK	DINNER
Raw vegetables—say 1 cup spinach, 1 cup lettuce, and 1 avocado, with red pepper for color; coconut water or nettle tea throughout the day	Walnuts, raspberries	Vegetable soup (make a large batch that will give you leftovers) —for example, Pumpkin Soup with a fresh red pepper
Steamed vegetables— broccoli, asparagus, yams or sweet potatoes, onions, spinach, etc.; for example, 1 baked sweet potato with 1 big steamed or baked onion, topped with 1 dash olive oil	Almonds, blueberries	Steamed broccoli and asparagus with chopped parsley or cilantro leaves and 1 splash olive oil and lemon
Vegetable soup—for example, Village Soup or Pumpkin Soup	Pecans, apples	Leafy vegetables lightly steamed or in soup, topped with pine nuts or pumpkin seeds
Baked sweet potato or squash and as much sprouted seeds and grain as possible—alfalfa, mung beans, black-eyed peas, and so on; or add 1 cup steamed or slow-cooked black-eyed beans to a salad of lettuce with avocado	Raw cashews berries	Leftover soup; or baked sweet potato with ginger, cilantro, and 1 small piece baked fresh fish

raw-veggie chopping. (See the shopping list in appendix C for a complete list of foods you'll need for the Release stage.) Most of my patients are amazed by how calm they feel and how clear their skin looks and feels after just a few days on this diet.

The Radiate Meal Plan

In the Radiate stage, you'll expand your repertoire of foods to a varied palette of tastes and colors that can be modified to delight and sustain you for the rest of your life. On the Radiate Meal Plan (see table 11), you'll use more olive and coconut oil, and you'll focus on broadening the range of antioxidant- and omega-3-rich anti-inflammatory foods. The result will be rich and satisfying meals that bring deep pleasure and satisfac-

My Mum's Voice: Moderation

My maternal grandfather died at ninety-two. His philosophy was what the ancient Greeks referred to as *pan metron ariston*—everything in moderation. He loved my grandmother, a beautiful woman who was tough and solid as a rock—the true head of the family. My maternal grandfather followed all the traditions of our faith, even fasting occasionally throughout the year. He walked a great deal and he died without ever having been seriously ill. My paternal grandfather was healthy as well—he died at the ripe old age of 115! He worked well into his old age and made love until he was ninety.

Don't you ever wonder why chronic illnesses such as heart disease and type 2 diabetes were not as common in the past as they are now? I believe the answer is incredibly simple: People once ate simple, nutrient-rich, whole foods and, in the case of my Greek ancestors, consumed more olive oil, fruit, and legumes, all of which are rich in beneficial minerals and trace elements.

tion while reducing inflammation and guarding against future food sensitivities.

MORE RADIATE MEAL CHOICES

I hope that the first week on the Radiate Meal Plan gave you a flavor of how your eating can keep you in Positive Feedback. You'll follow the Radiate way of eating for the rest of your days. At this stage, you can feel free to experiment with new combinations of foods. As long as you take care to avoid the Release foods listed in chapter 5, you should be in good territory. In addition, take the time to do the food reactivity testing described in the previous chapter (under "Reintroducing Reactive Foods"), to further tailor the Radiate way of eating to your body's unique needs. Tables 12 through 16 offer additional options that you can mix and match as you explore.

Positive Feedback Supplements

Recent studies have found that long-term supplement usage may lead to less-than-favorable health outcomes. Of particular concern are vitamin E and vitamin A in supplement form (rather than from food)—but even standard multivitamins are raising some red flags. If you have any health concerns, be especially careful. For example, many supplements feature high levels of iodine, which can be problematic for people with thyroid or parathyroid issues. Only two supplements have so many positive benefits that I recommend using them every day:

Vitamin D: Take 2,000 to 3,000 international units (IU) daily. (Note: If blood tests indicate that you're deficient, under a doctor's care consider taking one 50,000-IU capsule weekly for six weeks.)

Omega-3 fish oils: Take 1,000 milligrams (mg) twice a day, one capsule in the morning, one at night.

Table 11. **The Radiate Meal Plan**

DAY	UPON WAKING	BREAKFAST	SNACK
Monday	Warm water with juice of ½ lemon	Steamed apple with cinnamon and manuka honey, along with ½ cup porridge oats	Your choice of tea, with a single choice from the snack list in table 15
Tuesday	Warm water with juice of ½ lemon	½ cup goat's-milk yogurt with gluten-free granola	Your choice of tea, with a single choice from the table 15
Wednesday	Warm water with juice of ½ lemon	Omega Smoothie	Your choice of tea, with a single choice from the snack list in table 15
Thursday	Warm water with juice of ½ lemon	Nutty Smoothie	Your choice of tea, with a single, choice from the snack list in table 15
Friday	Warm water with juice of ½ lemon	2 ounces smoked salmon with olive oil, 1 slice gluten-free rye bread, and ½ cup fruit or 1 piece fruit, with ½ cup goat's-milk yogurt topped with 1 tablespoon ground flaxseed	Your choice of tea, with a single choice from the snack list in table 15
Saturday	Warm water with juice of ½ lemon and ½ cup goat's-milk yogurt	2 to 3 gluten-free pancakes with a little honey or topped with fresh blueberries and grated apples, with 1 tablespoon ground flaxseed	Your choice of tea, with a single choice from the snack list in table 15
Sunday	Warm water with juice of ½ lemon	½ cup spelt or steel-cut oat porridge made with almond or rice milk and a little honey, topped with 2 to 3 tablespoons nuts or seeds and 1 tablespoon ground flaxseed, served with ¼ cup sheep's-milk ricotta on the side once a week if desired (to increase protein)	Your choice of tea, with a single choice from the snack list in table 15

LUNCH	SNACK	DINNER
Egg-white omelet made with 3 eggs, 1 ounce feta cheese, and chives to taste, with 2 slices gluten-free rye bread or a small side salad	Your choice of tea, with a single choice from the snack list in table 15	Baked hake with olive oil, capers, fresh tomatoes, shallots, and coriander, along with vegetables (two types, any preparation)
Salad with 4 ounces chicken or turkey or 1 ounce feta, goat, mozzarella, or hard cheese, topped with lightly roasted pine nuts and 1 tablespoon (each) olive oil and lemon juice, with 1 piece fresh fruit	Your choice of tea, with a single choice from the snack list in table 15	Grilled Greek Burgers
4 ounces protein of your choice, with vegetable soup as desired	Your choice of tea, with a single choice from the snack list in table 15	4 to 5 ounces tuna or lean grass-fed meat (beef, turkey, veal, etc.), with vegetables or nonstarchy salad (as desired), ½ to 1 cup brown rice, and 1 piece fresh fruit
Salad with 4 ounces chicken or turkey or 1 ounce feta, goat, mozzarella, or hard cheese, topped with lightly roasted pine nuts and 1 tablespoon (each) olive oil and lemon juice, with 1 piece fresh fruit	Your choice of tea, with a single choice from the snack list in table 15	Sea Bass baked in the oven with ginger, topped with olive oil and lemon, with steamed spinach, green beans, or broccoli
1 to 2 cups tuna or chicken salad on kale and lettuce or on a slice of gluten-free rye bread, with of gluten-free rye bread, with	Your choice of tea, with a single choice from the snack list in table 15	Grilled red peppers with ½ cup feta or goat cheese, topped with 1 tablespoon pine nuts, a dash oregano, and 1 tablespoon olive oil, with 3½ ounces protein of your choice
Salad with 4 ounces chicken or turkey or 1 ounce feta, goat, mozzarella, or hard cheese, topped with lightly roasted pine nuts and 1 tablespoon (each) olive oil and lemon juice, with 1 piece fresh fruit	Your choice of tea, with a single choice from the snack list in table 15	Grilled salmon on bed of steamed spinach, with Sweet Potato Puree
4 ounces protein of your choice, with vegetable soup as desired	Your choice of tea, with a single choice from the snack list in table 15	Roast Chicken, with steamed green beans or broccoli

Table 12. **Smoothie Recipes**

Berry Smoothie
 1 handful blueberries
 1 kiwi
 1 slice pineapple
 1 cup unsweetened organic almond milk
 1 scoop Warrior Blend protein powder or egg white protein
 1 tablespoon Udo's Choice Ultimate Oil Blend or olive oil

Protein Shake
 1 scoop Warrior Blend protein powder
 2 teaspoons plain goat's-milk yogurt
 ½ banana
 1 kiwi
 7 blueberries or blackberries, or 1 peach, or ½ papaya, or 2 slices pineapple,
    or ½ pear with the seeds

Warrior Smoothie
 ½ to 1 cup plain yogurt
 ½ cup berries
 ½ banana
 1 teaspoon honey
  1 scoop Warrior Blend protein powder
 1 cup unsweetened organic almond milk (and ice if desired)

Nutty Smoothie
 1 cup plain goat's milk yogurt
 ½ to 1 cup blueberries, raspberries, or blackberries, or 1 peach, papaya, or pineapple
 2 to 3 tablespoons nuts of your choice
 1 tablespoon ground flaxseed
 1 tablespoon sunflower seeds
 1 tablespoon goji berries

Omega Smoothie
 1 handful blueberries, raspberries, or blackberries
 1 slice pineapple
 1 tablespoon Udo's Choice Ultimate Oil Blend or olive oil
 1 tablespoon ground flaxseed

Tropical Smoothie
 4 kiwi berries
 1 whole small organic lemon, peeled
 1 cup unsweetened organic almond milk or 1 scoop protein powder with vanilla taste
 ½ apple or pear
 2 slices pineapple
 1 tablespoon Udo's Choice Ultimate Oil Blend or olive oil

Table 12. **Smoothie Recipes** *(continued)*

Kiwi Lemon Smoothie

    1 kiwi

    7 blueberries or blackberries

    1 whole small organic lemon, peeled

    2 slices pineapple

    4 walnuts

    3 almonds

    1 tablespoon Udo's Choice Ultimate Oil Blend or olive oil

Almond Chocolate Smoothie

    1 scoop chocolate-flavored protein powder

    ½ banana

    1 kiwi

    1 whole small organic lemon, peeled

    1 tablespoon olive oil or coconut oil

    1 handful blueberries or blackberries

    1 tablespoon organic almond butter

    1 cup unsweetened organic almond milk

    3 walnuts

Kale Smoothie

    1 handful blueberries

    5 large kale leaves

    ½ banana

    1 cup unsweetened organic almond milk (and ice if desired)

    1 scoop Warrior Blend protein powder

    1 tablespoon almond butter

    1 tablespoon coconut oil

Table 13. **Additional Breakfast Options**

Egg-white omelet made with 2 or 3 eggs cooked in olive oil, with added goat or feta cheese and chopped tomato with thyme, with a side of steamed spinach

1 cup plain goat's-milk yogurt mixed with ½ to 1 cup fruit (blueberries, raspberries, blackberries, or pineapple chunks); 2 to 3 tablespoons unsalted walnuts or almonds; and 1 tablespoon goji berries

1 cup plain goat's-milk yogurt mixed with 1 peach or papaya; 1 tablespoon sunflower seeds or pumpkin seeds; and 1 tablespoon goji berries

2 to 3 boiled eggs (eating only the whites) drizzled with olive oil and sprinkled with sea salt and pepper to taste

2 ounces smoked or poached salmon with olive oil on 1 slice gluten-free rye bread, with ½ cup fruit (or 1 piece fruit) and 1 cup plain goat's-milk yogurt mixed with 1 tablespoon ground flaxseed

2 to 3 gluten-free pancakes with a little honey or Stevia sweetener, topped with fresh blueberries or grated apples

½ cup steel-cut oats or gluten-free organic oat porridge made with unsweetened almond milk, 1 tablespoon raw honey or manuka honey, 2 to 3 tablespoons nuts or seeds, and 1 tablespoon ground flaxseed; with ½ cup ricotta on the side once a week if desired (to increase protein)

½ cup steel-cut oats with 1 tablespoon goji berries and 1 tablespoon cocoa nibs (crumbled raw cacao beans)

Organic millet rice or oat bran–flake cereal (special treat!), with unsweetened organic almond milk or rice milk

2 slices wheat-free toasted bread drizzled with olive oil (or spread with almond butter) and topped with sliced avocado

2 to 3 slices roasted/steamed turkey (not smoked) on 1 slice wheat-free rye bread, with ½ cup fruit (or 1 apple or pear) and ½ cup plain yogurt mixed with 1 tablespoon pumpkin seeds or ground flaxseed

Table 14. **Additional Lunch or Dinner Options**

Best eaten about 12:30 P.M. and 6:30 P.M.

4 to 5 ounces lean protein (tuna, buffalo, turkey, veal, or grass-fed beef), 1 serving veggies or salad as desired (nonstarchy), and ½ to 1 cup brown rice, with ½ to 1 cup fruit (or 1 piece fruit)

1 to 2 cups tuna or chicken salad on kale and lettuce or on 1 slice gluten-free rye bread, with ½ to 1 cup fruit (or 1 piece fruit) or side salad

4 to 5 ounces protein of your choice

1 cup vegetable soup

California Fresh Salad with 4 to 5 ounces chicken or turkey and 1 ounce cheese (feta, goat, mozzarella, or hard cheese), topped with lightly roasted pine nuts, 1 tablespoon olive oil, and 1 tablespoon lemon juice, with ½ to 1 cup fruit (or 1 piece fruit)

Pan-Grilled Tuna (or Mahi-Mahi or Sea Bass), with grilled asparagus and broccoli

Toasted rye with olive oil and tomato and buffalo mozzerella with basil leaf

Table 15. **Snack Options**

Best at approximately 11:00 A.M. and 3:30 P.M.

1 ounce nuts (5 to 10) and 1 piece fruit

1 to 2 ounces (slices) cheese and fruit

1 wheat-free crust (available at Whole Foods)

1 2-percent Greek-style yogurt with 3 to 4 walnuts and 2 slices pineapple

2 to 3 gluten-free organic rice cakes with organic almond butter or sesame tahini or manuka or Greek honey (flavored with sage or thyme) or avocado

¼ to ⅓ cup nut/fruit mix (walnuts, almonds, prunes, figs)

¼ to ⅓ cup mix almonds, walnuts, goji berries, and dark-chocolate cocoa nibs

1 organic apple with 5 to 6 almonds

Ginger, lemon, and manuka honey tea with 1 teaspoon grated ginger and lemon juice

Table 16. **Special Treats**

Indulge only 1 to 2 times a week

Glass champagne

2 to 3 squares dark chocolate (greater than 75 percent cocoa)

1 shot high-quality tequila with fresh grapefruit juice

1 shot rye vodka

Table 17. **Healing Teas**

Chamomile

Dandelion

Echinacea

Ginger

Ginkgo biloba

Green

Hibiscus

Jasmine

Lemon balm

Milk thistle

Nettle

Oolong

Peppermint

Rooibos

Rosehip

White

Yerba Mate

8

The Positive Feedback Recipes

Preparing food and sharing it with loved ones is one of the most radiant experiences on earth. I recently moved to California, and my husband has been spoiling me with the most amazing fresh dinners, highlighting line-caught fish, truly fresh farmers' market vegetables, sweet berries, and crunchy salads with lemon and olive oil. Even if you don't live in California, your local grocery store has an entire produce section full of delights waiting for you. Shoot for a variety of vegetables every week; don't allow yourself to get into a rut. If it helps to keep things exciting, challenge yourself to try a new vegetable or fruit every week. Or sign up for a share in a CSA, shorthand for a local farm that sells weekly subscriptions—what's come to be known as "community supported agriculture." From what my friends tell me, there's no greater culinary challenge than using all your CSA vegetables in a week! That good pressure will help broaden your horizons, and the produce is often delivered straight to your door.

Whenever possible, use organic produce to reduce the toxins you ingest. Although it tends to be more expensive, it's well worth it. The same goes for cage-free and grass-fed poultry and meats. Not only are they better for you, but they taste better, too!

To inspire you, I've included in this chapter some of my absolute favorite recipes, collected over a lifetime of meals with my mother, Jenny, and my husband, Jerry, both amazing cooks who really know how to bake their love into everything they prepare for the family!

Salads

California Fresh Salad

SERVES 2 TO 3

> 3 cups iceberg lettuce, chopped
>
> 1 beef tomato chopped
>
> 1 cup ripe avocado, sliced
>
> ½ shallot, finely chopped
>
> ½ cup cilantro leaves, finely chopped
>
> ½ lime, juiced
>
> ½ lemon, juiced
>
> 2 tablespoons extra-virgin olive oil
>
> Sea salt and freshly ground pepper to taste
>
> ½ cup gluten-free tortilla chips

Combine the lettuce, tomatoes, and avocado in a large bowl. In a small bowl, whisk together the shallot, cilantro, lime juice, olive oil, and salt and/or pepper. Pour this dressing over the salad mixture and toss everything well. Sprinkle with tortilla chips just before serving.

(Optional: You can turn this salad into a main course by adding albacore tuna or leftovers from your roast chicken or turkey. Pair with short-grain brown rice or quinoa.)

Greek Goddess Salad

SERVES 2 TO 3

2 cups ripe tomatoes, chopped

1 cup Persian cucumbers, chopped

½ white onion, finely chopped

½ cup green olives

½ cup parsley, finely chopped

½ cup feta cheese (goat or sheep)

2 tablespoons extra-virgin olive oil

½ lemon, juiced

½ cup salted or unsalted capers

½ teaspoon dry oregano

Sea salt and freshly ground pepper to taste

Before prepping other vegetables, chop the onion and put it in water with 1 teaspoon salt to kill the onion's strong taste. Once all the other vegetables have been prepared, combine olives, tomatoes, cucumber, parsley, feta, and rinsed/drained onion in a large bowl. Toss with olive oil and lemon and top with capers. Sprinkle oregano and salt and pepper to taste.

Fresh Spinach Salad

SERVES 2 TO 3

1½ 6-ounce bags washed baby spinach

2 to 3 hardboiled eggs, peeled (yolks discarded) and chopped

½ cup pine nuts

2 tablespoons pomegranate seeds

2 tablespoons extra-virgin olive oil

Sea salt and freshly ground pepper to taste

Combine spinach, eggs, pine nuts, and pomegranate seeds in a large bowl. Drizzle the salad with olive oil right before serving, seasoning to taste.

Jerry's Crab Salad

SERVES 2

> 2 cups white crab meat
>
> ½ shallot, finely chopped
>
> 1 tablespoon lemongrass, finely chopped
>
> 1 teaspoon fresh grated ginger
>
> 1 tablespoon fresh basil leaves, finely chopped
>
> 1 lime, juiced
>
> 1 tablespoon purchased Thai fish sauce
>
> 1 tablespoon toasted sesame oil
>
> 1 head baby gem romaine lettuce, washed and separated
>
> ½ tablespoon Thai chili pepper (optional), seeded and finely chopped

Gently fold the crab meat, shallot, lemongrass, ginger, basil leaves, lime juice, fish sauce, and sesame oil in a bowl. Serve the romaine leaves, still whole, separately. At the table, scoop the crab mixture into individual leaves of romaine. Add chopped chili pepper if you can take the spice!

Fruit Salad

SERVES 4

> ½ cup ripe kiwi, peeled and cut into bite-size pieces
>
> ½ cup whole strawberries, stemmed
>
> ½ cup blueberries
>
> ½ cup raspberries
>
> ½ cup blackberries
>
> ½ lemon, juiced
>
> Stevia, to taste

This recipe can be made using any combination of fresh seasonal berries (2 to 2½ cups total). Gently toss kiwi, strawberries (left whole!), blueberries, raspberries, and blackberries with the lemon juice and Stevia sweetener. Let the mixture (covered) sit overnight in the refrigerator. Serve as is or with a spoonful of goat's-milk yogurt.

Soups

Pumpkin (or Sweet Potato) Soup

SERVES 4

> 4 cups pumpkin, peeled, seeded, and chopped (or 3 small sweet
>   potatoes, peeled and chopped)
> 1 cup red pepper, seeded and chopped
> 1 cup zucchini, chopped
> 1 cup yellow onions, chopped
> ½ cup celery with stem, chopped
> 6 to 7 tablespoons extra-virgin olive oil
> ½ cup toasted pumpkin seeds
> 1 cup crumbled goat cheese (or hard cheese)
> 2 teaspoons fresh grated ginger

Place the chopped pumpkin (or sweet potato), zucchini, onions and celery
in a large soup pot and add the vegetable stock until at least half the
vegetables are covered. Bring the broth to a boil then let simmer over
low heat for 30 minutes. Turn off the heat and let the soup cool to room
temperature before pureeing vegetable and broth in a blender. Add 2 to 3
tablespoons of olive oil to the pureed mixture and return the soup to the
pot and let simmer for 15 minutes before serving in individual soup bowls.
Top each serving with 1 tablespoon of olive oil and the pumpkin seeds,
crumbled cheese, and ginger.

Village Soup

SERVES 4

> 1 cup yellow onion, grated
> 1 cup carrots, sliced
> 1 cup celery, chopped
> 1 cup red pepper, chopped

1 cup ripe vine tomatoes (or 1 tablespoon tomato paste)

1 vegetable bouillon cube

3 to 4 cups water

2 tablespoons extra-virgin olive oil

Sea salt and freshly ground pepper to taste

Combine the onion, carrots, celery, red pepper, and tomatoes (or tomato paste), along with the bouillon cube, in a stockpot containing 3 to 4 cups water. Simmer the mixture on low heat for 30 minutes. Add the olive oil and seasoning just before serving.

Main Dishes

Oven-Baked Branzino with Cherry Tomato and Caper Salsa

SERVES 2

1 whole sea bass, skin and bones intact

Crystal sea salt flakes

½ cup flat-leaf parsley

1 lemon, half sliced for stuffing, half juiced for salsa

½ cup cherry tomatoes, stemmed

1 tablespoon shallot, finely diced

1 tablespoon salted Sicilian capers

2 to 3 tablespoons extra-virgin olive oil

Sea salt to taste

Preheat the oven to 375°F. Place sea bass in a baking dish or on an oven-safe tray. Salt both sides of the fish, as well as the cavity. Stuff the cavity with parsley stems and lemon slices. Bake the fish 15 to 20 minutes. (To check if the fish is cooked through, place a sharp knife through the thickest part of the flesh. If the tip of the blade is warm to the touch when removed, the fish should be ready to eat.) Remove the fish from the oven tray (to halt further cooking) and let it rest 4 to 5 minutes. Discard the parsley and lemon stuffing.

To prepare the salsa, quarter the cherry tomatoes and place in a small bowl with the shallot, capers, and lemon juice. Gently mix those ingredients; then add the olive oil and stir. If you prefer to use unsalted capers, you may want to add salt to taste.

Remove the skin from the baked sea bass and gently lift the fillets from the bone. Serve on a large plate with steamed vegetables (such as broccoli), which can be drizzled with olive oil and lemon for extra flavor. Garnish the fish with generous amounts of salsa. (Note: This recipe also works well with Alaskan halibut, Red Snapper or Grey Mullet.)

Pan-Grilled Ahi Tuna or Mahi-Mahi

SERVES 2 TO 3

1½ pounds fresh Ahi tuna or Mahi Mahi steaks

Sea salt and pepper to taste

2 to 3 tablespoons extra-virgin olive oil

1 tablespoon lemongrass, finely chopped

1 teaspoon fresh grated ginger

1 teaspoon fresh basil leaves, chopped

Rub olive oil on the tuna steaks and season both sides of the fish steaks with salt and pepper on both sides. For medium-rare, fry the fish in a hot pan for 5 to 6 minutes on each side (depending on the thickness of the steaks), turning over only once. The fish should be nicely browned on the outside but still pinkish on the inside. Add the lemongrass, ginger, and basil leaves to 2 to 3 tablespoons of olive oil and the lemon juice in a shallow bowl and stir. Season with a little salt and pepper. Let the mixture rest for at least 30 minutes before drizzling over the tuna steaks.

Butterflied Roast Chicken

SERVES 4 TO 6

  1 whole large chicken

  1 teaspoon garlic, finely chopped

  1 cup white sweet onion, thinly sliced

  2 to 3 tablespoons extra-virgin olive oil

  1 tablespoon freshly squeezed lemon juice

  1 teaspoon dry oregano

  Sea salt and freshly ground pepper to taste

Preheat the oven to 375°F. Using a sharp knife, split the chicken down the back and remove the backbone. Stuff garlic between the skin and the breast meat for flavor and season both sides of the chicken with salt and pepper. Lay the onion slices in a baking pan that has been greased with a little olive oil. Place the flattened chicken halves on top of the onion, skin side up. Drizzle with olive oil and season with oregano. Roast the chicken for 1½ hours, until the skin is golden brown. To check if the chicken is thoroughly cooked, place a skewer or a sharp knife into the thickest part of the thigh and remove. If the tip of the skewer or knife is warm to the touch, the chicken is ready to be removed from the oven. Take the pan out and pour the lemon juice onto the sizzling skin. Let the chicken rest for 10 to 15 minutes before carving and serving..

Egg-White Frittata with Feta Cheese and Chives

SERVES 1

  3 eggs (whites only)

  ¼ cup goat's-milk feta cheese

  ½ tablespoon bunch chives, finely snipped

  1 tablespoon extra-virgin olive oil

Place the egg whites in a mixing bowl, discarding the yolks. Crumble the feta into the bowl, add the chives, and mix well. Heat the olive oil in a large frying pan over medium heat. Add the egg mixture, which will form a thin bubbly layer on the base of the pan. Remove the pan from the heat when a golden crust forms around the edges of the frittata and the center seems fully cooked. Slide the frittata onto a large plate. Serve with a slice of toasted 100-percent rye bread or a tomato and red onion salad.

Cabrito with Prunes

SERVES 4

> **2 large Cabrito goat thighs cut into 3-inch-long pieces**
> **3 cups white/yellow onions, sliced**
> **1 tablespoon dry oregano**
> **1 cup vegetable stock**
> **1 tablespoon garlic, finely chopped**
> **1 cup freshly squeezed lemon juice**
> **2 cups seedless prunes**
> **Sea salt and freshly ground pepper to taste**
> **½ cup olive oil**

Place the pieces of Cabrito, onions, oregano, vegetable stock, garlic, lemon juice, prunes, and salt and pepper in a Dutch oven or other stovetop pan. Bring the liquid to a boil then turn down the heat and leave to cook on a medium-low setting. Stir the meat around after 1 hour and continue cooking over low heat until vegetables are tender and the liquid has been reduced by about half (about 90 minutes to 2 hours). Plate the Cabrito pieces with vegetables and drizzle a little olive oil at the end to give the meat a nice sheen. This dish is delicious on its own or accompanied with brown rice, quinoa, or pearl barley.

Roast Chicken/Turkey with Figs

SERVES 4 TO 6

4 to 6 dried rosemary sprigs

4 cups chicken thighs or breasts or turkey breasts

2 cups yellow onions, sliced

8 to 10 figs

1 clove garlic, finely chopped

1 cup vegetable stock

1 pinch dry oregano

1 lemon, juiced

2 to 3 tablespoons extra-virgin olive oil

Sea salt and freshly ground pepper to taste

Preheat the oven to 350°F. Place the chicken or turkey pieces on top of the rosemary sprigs in a baking dish that has been greased with a little olive oil. Roast the meat in the oven for 60 minutes, turning occasionally until brown. Remove the pan from the oven and add onion, figs, garlic, vegetable stock, oregano, lemon juice, olive oil, and salt and pepper. Place the tray back in the oven for an additional 30 minutes before removing and serving.

Jenny's Greek Bolognese Sauce

SERVES 4 TO 6

2 pounds lean ground beef

2 cups white/yellow onions

4 cups ripe vine tomatoes (blended into juice)

2 bay leaves

2 cinnamon sticks

1 teaspoon cinnamon

1 whole carrot, peeled

1 cup vegetable stock

3 to 4 tablespoons extra-virgin olive oil

Sea salt and pepper to taste

Brown the meat over medium heat in a large saucepan. Grate in the onions and add the tomato juice, bay leaves, cinnamon sticks, cinnamon, carrot, and vegetable stock. Season with salt and pepper to taste. Stir until all the ingredients are mixed well. Cover the saucepan and cook over low heat, for 45 to 60 minutes. Turn off the burner and let the sauce rest and cool for 10 minutes before adding olive oil. Serve with gluten-free spaghetti.

Greek Burgers

SERVES 4

4 cups lean ground beef or turkey

1 bunch parsley, finely chopped

½ tablespoon dry oregano

1 cup vegetable stock

1 large white onion, grated

2 tablespoons extra-virgin olive oil

1 egg

1 slice gluten-free rye bread

Sea salt and freshly ground pepper to taste

Preheat the oven to 350°F. Place the rye bread in a bowl of hot water for 2 to 3 minutes to soften. Combine the meat, parsley, oregano, vegetable stock, onion, olive oil, egg, bread, salt, and pepper in a large mixing bowl. Separate the mixture into ½-inch, palm-size patties. Arrange the patties on a baking tray that has been greased with a little olive oil and bake for 20 to 25 minutes, until golden brown. (Note: Serve with slice of feta drizzled with olive oil and pair with Greek Goddess Salad.)

Mediterranean Salsa (for Fish)

SERVES 2

> 1 shallot, finely chopped
>
> 3 mini–sweet peppers (red, orange, and yellow), finely chopped
>
> 1 tomato, finely chopped
>
> ½ tablespoon garlic, finely chopped
>
> ½ tablespoon cilantro leaves, finely chopped
>
> ½ cup almond-stuffed olives, thinly sliced
>
> 1 tablespoon freshly squeezed lime juice
>
> 1 tablespoon freshly squeezed lemon juice
>
> 3 tablespoons extra-virgin olive oil
>
> Sea salt and freshly ground pepper to taste

Mix the shallot, peppers, tomato, garlic, cilantro, olives, lemon and lime juice, and olive oil. Leave the mixture to rest for a least 1 hour at room temperature. Sample at that point and add salt and pepper to taste. This salsa is delicious served with a whole roasted fish or with grilled tuna or mahi-mahi steaks.

Side Dishes

Speltotto (Pearled-Spelt Risotto)

SERVES 4

> 4 cups vegetable stock (recipe below), hot
>
> 2 cups pearled spelt
>
> 2 leeks
>
> 4 cups kale (a mixture of Russian, English, and Tuscan works well)
>
> ¼ cup unsalted butter
>
> 1 tablespoon olive oil
>
> ½ cup shallots, finely chopped
>
> 1 cup grated hard goat cheese

FOR THE VEGETABLE STOCK:

2 tablespoons extra-virgin olive oil

1 cup yellow onion, grated

2 cups carrots, peeled and grated

1 tablespoon garlic, minced

2 cups celery, finely chopped

2 bay leaves

5 cups boiling water

DIRECTIONS FOR THE STOCK:

Sauté the garlic, onions, and grated carrots in a saucepan over medium-low heat for 2 minutes taking care not to brown them; then add bay leaves and 5 cups boiling water. Return the mixture to a boil and simmer for 10 minutes. Strain to create the vegetable stock—a "light vegetable tea"—which is now ready to be used for the risotto.

DIRECTIONS FOR THE PEARLED SPELT RISOTTO:

Place the spelt in a sieve, rinse it under the cold tap, and then soak it in a bowl of cold water for 15 minutes. While it's soaking, halve the leeks lengthwise, rinse carefully, and chop finely. Strip the leaves from the stalks (or spines) of the kale and roughly chop the leaves. Set aside the leeks and kale.

Stir for a couple minutes, making sure that all the grains are well coated and not sticking together. Using a ladle, gradually add the hot stock in batches, stirring frequently until the liquid is absorbed before ladling in more stock. Repeat this step until the spelt is almost cooked through. (This will take about 20 minutes. You may not need all the stock.) Add the kale and cook for a further 2 to 3 minutes. Stir in the butter and half the cheese. In a large saucepan over low heat, gently sauté the shallots without browning them. After a couple minutes, add the leeks and cook for a further 2 to 3 minutes. Again, be very careful not to brown the vegetables. They need to be translucent.

Drain the spelt well and add to the pan with the leeks and shallots. Garnish individual servings with the remaining cheese.

A salad of baby leaves makes a good side. (Kale, chard, and beetroot leaves work well with this dish.)

(Note: Spelt contains more protein and fiber than rice does, and is more filling. In order to make this a light dish, it's important to use a greater ratio of vegetables to grains than you would in a normal risotto.)

Short-Grain Brown Rice or Quinoa

SERVES 2 TO 3

> 2 cups water
> 1 cup vegetable stock
> 3 to 4 tablespoons extra-virgin olive oil
> ½ lemon, juiced
> 1 cup brown rice or quinoa

In a large saucepan, bring the water to a boil on high heat. Add the vegetable stock, olive oil, and lemon juice. When the mixture comes to a boil again, add the brown rice or quinoa, lower the heat, and let the mixture simmer, covered, for 35 minutes. Serve with California Fresh Salad or raw or steamed vegetables.

Spinach and Rice

SERVES 2 TO 3

> ½ cup spring (green) onion, chopped
> 5 cups fresh spinach, washed, drained, and chopped
> 6½ cups water
> 1⅓ cups short-grain brown rice
> 1 lemon, juiced (about 2 tablespoons)
> ⅓ cup extra-virgin olive oil
> Sea salt and freshly ground pepper

In a stockpot, fry the spring onion in 1 tablespoon of olive oil over medium heat for 2 to 3 minutes. Add the spinach and 1⅓ cups water and cook until the spinach wilts, about 5 to 7 minutes. Add the rice and remaining 5¼ cups water; bring the mixture to a boil and let it simmer, uncovered, for 15 minutes, stirring occasionally. Stir in the lemon juice; cook for another 5 minutes and then remove the pan from the heat. Stir in the remaining olive oil and cover the pan. Let the dish sit for 20 minutes until the ingredients "meld." Season with salt and pepper to taste.

This delicious traditional dish is a warming and hearty meal in itself, or it can be served as a side dish with a light entrée. Try topping it with a sprinkle of crumbled sheep's-milk feta.

Steamed Asparagus with Lemon

SERVES 2 TO 3

1 bunch asparagus
2 to 3 tablespoons extra-virgin olive oil
½ lemon, juiced
Sea salt and freshly ground pepper to taste

Break off the tough lower portion of each asparagus stalk. Cook the asparagus in a covered steamer over medium heat until al dente (that is, firm but not hard), about 5 to 6 minutes. Plate the cooked asparagus and drizzle it with the olive oil and lemon juice. Add sea salt and pepper to taste.

Garlic and Chili Broccolini (Long-Stem Broccoli)

SERVES 2 TO 3

5 to 7 long stems broccolini
1 clove garlic, finely chopped
1 small red chili, finely chopped

½ **lemon, juiced**

1 tablespoon extra-virgin olive oil

Sea salt and pepper to taste

Cook the broccolini in a covered steamer over medium heat until tender (about 5 to 6 minutes). Remove the broccolini and place in a shallow bowl on top of the garlic; this cooks the garlic slightly and cuts the bite. Prepare the dressing by whisking together the lemon juice and olive oil in a small bowl; add salt and pepper to taste. After the broccolini have cooled slightly but remain warm, pour on the dressing and toss to coat them evenly. Serve warm.

French Green Beans

SERVES 4 TO 6

4 cups fresh thin green beans

1 cup flat parsley leaves, thinly chopped

2 cups sweet potato, peeled and roughly chopped

2 cups large yellow onions, thinly sliced

1 cup zucchini, thinly sliced

3 cups ripe vine tomatoes, juiced in blender

2 cups vegetable stock

3 to 4 tablespoons extra-virgin olive oil

Place the beans, parsley, sweet potato, onions, and zucchini in a big stockpot. Add the tomato juice and the vegetable stock. Bring to a boil on medium heat; then simmer for 45 minutes on very low heat, until the vegetables are soft and most of the liquid has been absorbed. Add 3 to 4 tablespoons extra-virgin olive oil after you turn off the burner. Let the dish rest and cool for 15 minutes, then serve.

Black-Eyed Peas

SERVES 2 TO 3

  2 cups dry black-eyed peas

  1 large tomato, finely chopped

  1 large sweet white onion, finely chopped

  1 cup parsley, chopped

  ½ lemon, juiced

  2 to 3 tablespoons extra-virgin olive oil

Begin this recipe a day in advance. Place the peas in a pot with enough water to cover the peas. Bring the liquid to a boil then turn off the burner and let the peas sit in the hot water for 1 hour. Drain, then add fresh water and leave the peas soaking overnight.

Drain the peas before cooking them in a covered steamer over medium heat for 15 minutes. Place them in a large serving bowl. Add the onion, tomato, parsley, lemon juice, and olive oil and mix gently. Serve while still warm.

Peas and Artichoke Hearts

SERVES 4 TO 5

  2 cups fresh (or frozen) garden peas, shelled

  10 canned or frozen artichoke hearts

  1 cup yellow onion, chopped

  ½ cup spring (green) onions, thinly sliced

  ½ cup fresh dill, finely chopped

  1 cup vegetable stock

  ½ lemon, juiced

  2 to 3 tablespoons extra-virgin olive oil

  Sea salt and freshly ground pepper to taste

Place the peas, artichoke hearts, onion (both types), and dill in a large saucepan. Add the vegetable stock and simmer, covered, for 30 minutes. Remove the pan from the heat and add the olive oil and lemon juice, along with salt and pepper to taste. Let the dish rest 15 minutes before serving.

White Beans with Cinnamon

SERVES 2 TO 3

2 cups dry white beans

1 cup yellow onion, finely chopped

½ cup fresh parsley flat leaves, finely chopped

1 cup ripe vine tomato, thinly sliced

1 cinnamon stick

1 cup vegetable stock

2 tablespoons extra-virgin olive oil

Sea salt and freshly ground pepper to taste

Begin this recipe a day in advance. Place the beans in a pot with enough water to cover the beans. Bring the liquid to a boil then turn off the burner and let the beans sit in the hot water for 1 hour. Drain, then add fresh water and leave the beans soaking overnight.

Drain the beans and put them in a large stockpot. Add the onion, parsley, tomato, and cinnamon stick. Pour in the vegetable stock and simmer the mixture on low heat for 5 minutes. Just prior to serving, remove the cinnamon stick and add the olive oil, along with salt and pepper to taste.

Sweet Potato Mash

SERVES 4

3 cups sweet potatoes

1 handful cilantro, finely chopped

2 teaspoons fresh grated ginger

2 tablespoons extra-virgin olive oil

1 sprig coriander (optional)

Preheat the oven to 400°F. Place the sweet potatoes on a baking tray and bake for 1 hour. Remove the potatoes and set aside for 15 minutes to cool. Split potatoes in half with a knife and scoop out the flesh into a mixing bowl with the cilantro, ginger, and olive oil. Mix well until the consistency of the mash is to the desired smoothness. Serve with a drizzle of olive oil and a sprig of coriander (if desired).

Chickpea Salad

SERVES 2 TO 3

½ cup pine nuts

2 cups canned chickpeas

2 cloves garlic, finely chopped

1 teaspoon lemon juice

½ teaspoon cumin

½ teaspoon cinnamon

Sea salt to taste

1 tablespoon olive oil

½ teaspoon finely chopped parsley

Place the pine nuts in a dry skillet and cook over medium-low heat until they are golden-brown. They burn easily, so stir often (and remove them from the pan immediately after cooking). Warm the chickpeas in a pan with water. Drain them and transfer to a serving bowl. Gently mix in the

toasted pine nuts, garlic, lemon juice, cumin, and cinnamon. Season to
taste with salt. Top with a drizzle of olive oil and garnish with parsley.

Note: You can use dry chickpeas if you prefer. In that case, begin this
recipe a day in advance. Place the chickpeas in a pot with enough water
to cover the chickpeas. Bring the liquid to a boil then turn off the burner
and let the chickpeas sit in the hot water for an hour. Drain, then add fresh
water and leave the chickpeas soaking overnight. Drain them again before
continuing with the recipe as written.

Guacamole

SERVES 4 TO 6

5 avocados

3 mini–sweet peppers, finely chopped

2 tomatoes, seeded and then diced

1 big white onion, finely chopped

2 to 3 tablespoons finely chopped cilantro

Sea salt and freshly ground pepper to taste

Cut the avocadoes in half and discard the pits. Scoop out the avocado
"flesh" into a mixing bowl. Using a fork, mash the avocado to the desired
consistency. Add the peppers, tomatoes, onion, and cilantro and combine
gently. Season with salt and pepper to taste; then transfer to a serving dish.

9

The Positive Feedback Remedies

As most osteopaths in Britain do, I spend a great deal of one-on-one time with my patients, going over their entire medical history, their family history, and their current life stresses. I delve as far as feels comfortable for the patient, because the more information I have, the better I can develop what doctors call a "differential diagnosis"—a patient-centered approach that examines all the physical and emotional evidence to see what's *really* going on, not just what seems on the surface to be going on. What emotional pain are you suppressing that is now manifesting in a physical way?

That sore throat you had on vacation—that you didn't want to disrupt the family trip to go to the doctor for and promptly "forgot" about thereafter—could reveal itself to be something that needs immediate attention, such as a parathyroid nodule or cyst.

Most often, however, the diagnosis is not so dire, and the remedy is not invasive surgery. Instead, the remedies I prescribe most often are slight tweaks to the combination of meditation/introspection exercises, dietary changes, and exercise prescriptions that I suggest in the Positive Feedback core program.

I've created a mini–remedy plan for some of the most common issues that can be treated with self-help techniques—and, in certain cases, some clear guidelines about when you *must* see a doctor.

ANGER

Self-Healing Trigger Points:

> Focus on front-body points B, E, and M as well as back-body points D and G.

Other Remedies:

- Nine-point meditation

- The Tibetan Rites of Rejuvenation poses

- Positive Feedback meditation

- Vigorous exercise

- Talking with a loved one to release the anger or have a good cry

- Quiet, calm, and peace (e.g., avoiding idle chatter on the phone)

- Liver Flush cleanse (3 days)

- Give your physical and emotional house a good, deep cleaning. Toss anything that no longer works for you (including old relationships!)

- Lots of hugs and making love will unblock the pelvic area and move the Angry Liver energy toward balance and harmony.

ANXIETY AND DEPRESSION

Self-Healing Trigger Points:

> Focus on back-body points C, D, F, and G, as well as back-foot points M, N, and O.

Other Remedies:

Of the remedies listed below, those that are *products* (as opposed to processes) are available in various forms—bath oils, candles, room sprays. The oils for depression are as diverse as the ways in which depression manifests itself. Use whichever form most appeals to you—what's most important is the immediate feel it gives you, in the moment you need it most.

- Lavender (relaxing)

- Chamomile (good for sleep)

- Sandalwood (to increase feelings of safety and security; incense helps you clear "bad energy")

- Clary sage (good in bath)

- Ylang-ylang (good in bath)

- Bergamot (very uplifting lemon scent)

- Neroli (good for anxiety; helpful to pregnant moms)

- Natrum mur (homeopathic; especially useful if you are depressed and feeling sensitive but trying not to show it)

- Jasmine (increases confidence)

- Aconite (homeopathic; for extreme fear or trauma)

- Bach flower remedy (energizing)

- Fifteen- to twenty-minute bath in warm tub with 1 pound Epsom salts and 1 pound baking soda; plenty of rest afterward

- Time in the sunshine (increase that vitamin D!)

- Meditation exercises, focusing attention on the "third eye" (the point on your forehead above the bridge of your nose, between your two eyes)

- Extra baths (three during the Reflect week and three during the Release week)

COLDS AND COUGHS

Self-Healing Trigger Points:

> Work on front-body points C, D, L, M, and N combined with back-body points A, B, C, D, E, F, and G.

Other Remedies:

- Garlic (with parsley to kill the taste)

- Lemon water

- Hot steam (or inhaler) with therapeutic oils:

  - Lavender

  - Eucalyptus

  - Frankincense

  - Sandalwood

  - Tea tree

  - Peppermint

  - Rosemary

FLU

- Adrenoplex capsules (or other adrenal-supporting compounds of vitamins, minerals, and herbs)

- Oscillococcinum

- Hot baths

- Oregano-leaf "tea"

- Almond milk (no dairy)

HANGOVER

Self-Healing Trigger Points:

> Start with back-body leg and foot points, going from J to K to L to
> M, N, and O to reduce heat; continue on to points F and G to help
> the gut and large intestine, which are dehydrated and overworked;
> then do C and D to let go of sadness and grief and open up the
> heart; continue on to front-body points L and M for releasing the
> liver and stomach; and finally do G (heart protector) and B to
> calm the mind.

Other Remedies:

- Don't mix different alcohols (and alternate with water)

- Stick to champagne or wine, or look for spirits made from
  nonreactive sources (such as rye vodka or almond tequila; always
  order spirits on the rocks, to increase water intake)

- Vitamin B complex (take 1 at night before bed)

- Vitamin C (take 1 at night before bed)

- Nux vomica 30c (stops nausea; take 1 before bed and 1 in the
  morning)

- Calcium, magnesium, and vitamin C blend (e.g., Calma-C; take 1
  at night before bed)

- Coconut water or Smart water (to rehydrate and replenish
  electrolytes)

- Bananas (good source of potassium; also a natural antacid because
  they're high in magnesium, which can also help relax blood vessels
  to ease throbbing headaches)

- Almond butter, manuka honey, and banana sandwich on rye, topped with goji berries

- Probiotic mints (to kill mouth bacteria, for fresher morning breath!)

HEADACHE

Self-Healing Trigger Points:

> Start by first releasing back-body points A, B, C, D, E, F, and G, then M, N, and O. Continue with front-body points A, B, and C, and finish with top-of-foot points M and N.

Other Remedies:

- Realignment of vertebral spine (by chiropractor to encourage bloodflow)

- Orthotics in shoes (flat feet or heels all day can cause headaches)

- Allergy testing for food sensitivities—common for those with headaches: wheat, chocolate, milk/dairy, sulfites, sugar, citrus fruits (especially oranges and tangerines; grapefruit is better), fermented foods, vinegar, alcohol, MSG, chicken, cheese and sour cream, peanut butter, pork, and fresh-baked yeast products

- Chamomile colonic or coffee enema (if also constipated)

- CoQ10 coenzyme, 30 mg twice daily (for increased oxygenation)

- Calcium/magnesium before bed

- Blood test for anemia or vitamin B_6 deficiency

- Well-balanced diet supplemented by daily multivitamin and 1,000 mg vitamin C, with 1,000 mg fish oil twice daily

- Lavender oil (3 drops rubbed on temples or used on a cold compress on the forehead or back of neck at night)

- Peppermint oil (morning)

- Eucalyptus (good for sinus headache)

- Rosemary oil (if headache was caused by mucus and sinus infection)

- Arnica (if headache was caused by a bump on the head, to reduce trauma and speed healing)

- Belladonna (for fever-related headache)

- Pulsatilla tablets (for overwork, neuralgia)

- Sepia (for menstrual headache)

- Nux vomica (for headache with irritability, anger, or overwork)

- Natrum mur (all of the above, and migraines, especially when face is pale)

LOW BACK PAIN

Self-Healing Trigger Points:

> Start by first releasing back-body points C, D, E, F, H, I, J, K, and L. Continue with front-body points E, F, H, I, J, K, L, and M.

Other Remedies:

- Alternate hot and cold on pain (start with ice for 20 minutes, then hot bath for 20 minutes, with extra Epsom salts (2 to 3 packages); then ice pack for 20; then heating pad for 20; then ice pack—always end with cold!)

- If Epsom salts bath is in the morning, add peppermint oil or lavender oil (for calming energy); if in the evening, add lavender and chamomile (to help with sleep)

- Lower back massage (or lower back acupuncture or cranial sacral work)

- Lower back stabilizer

- Kinesiology tape over painful area (lifts the layer of skin/tissue over the sore muscles, to allow for increased oxygen and bloodflow to the area)

- Release meditations

- No alcohol!

- If acute, ask your doctor about anti-inflammatory medication to manage the pain

- If chronic, tell your doctor and your gynecologist about the pain during your annual exams (if standard tests are fine, but pain persists, consider having an ultrasound to rule out any other issues)

LOW LIBIDO

Self-Healing Trigger Points:

Focus on back-body points C, G, and F, then I, J, K, L, M, N, and O. Move on to front-body points B, C, D, G, H, I, M, and N.

Other Remedies:

- Jasmine (relaxing)

- Sandalwood (relaxing)

- Lower back massage (or lower back acupuncture or cranial sacral work)

- Rose mixed with lavender and few drops of ylang-ylang

- Black pepper with lavender

- Frankincense (1 drop in sweet almond oil)

- Patchouli

- Kegel exercises (all day long!)

- Pelvic tilt exercises (Tibetan pose #2)

MENSTRUAL PAIN

Self-Healing Trigger Points:

> You'll want to work on front-body points E, F, G, H, K, and M
> combined with back-body points C, D, E, H, I, J, K, L, M, N, and
> O. *Note:* Working on back-point K, on the *inside* of the ankle,
> helps release the deep inner muscles of the pelvis, which affect the
> sacroiliac area and the uterus; working at that same point, on the
> *outside* of the ankle, helps release any swelling of the outer gluteal
> muscles and the ovaries. (Note: Back K will also help men with
> their prostrate.)

Other Remedies:

- Use menstruation as a time of reflection on the completely
  intertwined nature of physical and emotional pain (also, celebrate
  this monthly reminder of your ability to give birth!)

- Increased protein (every meal, especially nuts, seeds, eggs, fish,
  and lean meats)

- Avoidance of sugar

- More hugs, love, and patience from loved ones (even "warning"
  your husband or boyfriend of your cycle, so they can understand
  and help)

- Avoidance of phosphates, coffee, and caffeinated drinks (which
  affect calcium absorption)

- Vitamin D

- Adequate fat in diet (low- or no-fat diet can increase mood swings;
  increase omega-3s to counter inflammation)

- Nutrient-rich diet—full of antioxidants to boost immune system

- Ample whole grains (brown rice, millet, oatmeal, quinoa, buckwheat) to balance hormones

- Arnica (pain relief, anti-inflammatory)

- Rhus tox (pain relief, anti-inflammatory)

- Get to know your cycle by tracking your periods in your calendar (helpful not only for you—especially when you want to get pregnant—but also good info to share with your doctor)

NECK PAIN

Self-Healing Trigger Points:

Start by first releasing back-body points A, B, C, D, M, N, and O. Continue with front-body points A, B, C, and D.

Other Remedies:

- Alternate hot and cold on pain (start with ice for 20 minutes, then hot bath for 20 minutes, with extra Epsom salts (2 to 3 packages); then ice pack for 20; then heating pad for 20; then ice pack—always end with cold!)

- If Epsom salts bath is in the morning, add peppermint oil or lavender oil (for calming energy); if in the evening, add lavender and chamomile (to help with sleep)

- Hot shower, holding 1.5 pound weight straight down, in the hand on the side with the pain

- Epsom salts baths

- Kinesiology tape over painful area (lifts the layer of skin/tissue over the sore muscles, to allow for increased oxygen and bloodflow to the area)

- Ensure that air conditioning is not too cold

- Release meditations

- No alcohol!

- If acute, ask your doctor about anti-inflammatory medication to manage the pain

- If chronic, check with your doctor or endocrinologist about thyroid testing (if blood tests are fine, consider having an ultrasound on the thyroid/parathyroid to rule out any other issues)

SORE THROAT

- Oregano-leaf "tea" (boil oregano leaves in water)

- Thyme oil / thyme tea (alternate oregano and thyme tea, 2 to 3 cups of each per day)

- Warm water with lemon (6 to 8 cups per day)

- Olive oil spray

- Bee pollen

- Manuka honey

- Balsam fir oil

- Thieves Oil (a Young Living product; massage on your chest in the bath, dilute it in the water, wear it on your skin in a steam room, or combine with sweet almond oil or grapeseed oil for a massage treatment)

- Marjoram oil bath (helpful with shivers and body aches)

- Lavender bath (to help you sleep, which is always the best remedy)

- Rosemary or peppermint (in the morning, as they are both stimulants)

- Fresh royal jelly (a little spoonful under the tongue)

THYROID

Self-Healing Trigger Points:

> Back-body point M on the middle and toward the outside of the toe will help in combination with the back-body points N to O.

Other Remedies:

- Pay close attention to odd symptoms—if you have any of these, see a doctor (preferably an endocrinologist) right away for a thyroid/parathyroid checkup:

- Neck pain, sore throat, or change in your voice ("losing" your voice)

- Sensitivity to cold, shivering, cold at night

- Fatigue (even if you've slept twelve hours)

- Jaw pain

- Gray tone in face

- Pain, tingling sensation around mouth and lips

- Dizziness, disorientation (feels like jetlag or exhaustion)

- Increased bowel movements

- Snappy, anxious, quick to anger

- A little dry, hard, yellow skin patch under your big toe and close to the ball of the foot

- Flaky nails, hair loss

- Palpitations, depression (especially during menstruation)

TRAVEL

Self-Healing Trigger Points:

> The points that really help with jet lag are front-body points A, B, C, D, G, and L and M. Massage each for ten seconds five times each while you're on the plane. If you can't sleep at night in your changed time zone, do that same collection of points and continue with back-body points F and G and N and O.

Other Remedies:

- Empty hotel fridge and fill it with items from the local health food store (one in every town)

- Get a full supply of fruit, goat's-milk yogurt, and other healthy snacks

- Bring your own pillow (I never travel without my TempurPedic pillow!)

- Redo Reflect exercises

- Maintain openness to adventure (every journey opens another door—enjoy it instead of dreading it)

- Opt for manual pat-down instead of machine scan at airport

- Request gluten-free meals or fruit platters on plane (see additional food suggestions, below)

- Use any time when you cannot sleep to write lists or notes, listen to music

- Resynchronize bedtime to local time

- Take a walk as soon as you arrive

- Water with lemon constantly (on plane, as soon as you land, in restaurants)

- Peppermint or green tea

- Multivitamins and/or vitamin C and omega-3s

- Dry brushing (especially if you never get a chance at home!)

- Request egg whites for face mask

- Hot bath with Epsom salts (15 to 20 minutes)

- Arnica

- Cocculus

- Nux vomica

- Melatonin

- Immune-defense spray, oregano oil/olive oil spray

- Bach rescue remedy spray

- Peppermint oil (three to four drops applied to the chest when you wake up)

- Lavender or chamomile (three to four drops applied to the chest at night)

- Wait 2 days before weighing yourself (travel can add 2 to 3 pounds of water retention)

Dietary Suggestions:

- Light meals, especially for the first few days, to help your body adjust (no sugar, wheat, or dairy)

- Emphasis on soups, salads, steamed spinach or other vegetables, fruit, fresh fish

- Big salad starter; no breads or desserts

- Breakfasts that support long days: gluten-free muesli with almond milk (or goat's milk or yogurt); cooked rolled oats with berries/

walnuts or warm apple and cinnamon; egg-white scrambled or poached eggs (with roast tomatoes, spinach, or sliced avocado instead of bread)

- Fruits that remedy traveler's digestive issues: kiwi, prunes, and figs (supply vitamin C, are good for bowels); pineapple and papaya (are anti-inflammatory, help with digestion and bowel function)

- Snacks keep energy up for long days: protein powder (two scoops with almond milk or water); goat's-milk yogurt with acidophilus, blueberries

The Positive Feedback Questionnaire

Because I don't have the honor of treating you directly, I'm going to provide you with a list of questions you can ask yourself about your own health. Take your time as you go through this list. Perhaps start a new journal, with the answers to these questions taking up the first ten or so pages. By the end of this questionnaire, you'll have a comprehensive collection of important factors impacting your health. Many people find that seeing these issues in black and white—taking them out of the darkness, out of denial—helps spur them to seek treatment. I hope that will be the case for you, too.

When I first meet with a client in my practice, I ask a series of questions that help me classify his or her pain by determining the following:

1. Whether it's acute or chronic pain

2. The specific area of the body involved

3. The system whose dysfunction may be causing the pain (e.g., nervous system, gastrointestinal system, dental structure)

4. The *presumed* reason for the pain

5. Whether the pattern has caused or was caused by abnormal function (e.g., decreased range of movement, headache, fibromyalgia, inflammation)

As you may recall from chapter 1, I've found that most people who come to me for help suffer from one of two types of back pain: lower back pain or upper back pain. Despite any additional health concerns—and most patients have some—one's back pain type is a potent diagnostic tool. As noted earlier, that body type suggests a constellation not only of physical symptoms, but of emotional and spiritual issues as well.

So what is *your* back pain type? The answers you give to the questions in table 18 will give you that answer. Set aside at least twenty minutes to take stock, quietly and reflectively, of the current state of your body. The questionnaire is quite lengthy by design: I want you to see just how many of your health concerns might be related to your back pain.

You'll see that the questions are presented in two columns. On the left are symptoms typically associated with upper back pain; on the right, lower back pain. Put a checkmark next to all those questions, regardless of column, to which you answer yes. When you get to the end, tally up your totals. The column with the highest number likely corresponds to your type.

While this is clearly not a medical diagnosis, it can be reassuring to know that you are not alone in your particular constellation of ailments—that many others share your same struggles. And best of all—*there is a way out of your pain.*

Please note, though: This questionnaire can only help guide you to understand your body's pain. For a full look at your current condition, you *must* consult with your medical practitioner, so he or she can rule out any serious concerns. Specifically, any tingling, numbness, or lack of sensation can be associated with a serious medical condition or disease. Even without such symptoms, when your pain is chronic or particularly intense, seek medical advice.

Table 18. **What's Your Back Pain Type?**

TYPE A – UPPER BACK PAIN	✓	TYPE B – LOWER BACK PAIN	✓
Do you get left or right shoulder pain?		Do you get lower back pain and hip pain?	
Do you get pain in your upper neck and back?		Are you generally tired?	
		Do you get constipated?	
Does your skin have a gray/blue tinge?		Do you get sick often?	
Are you stiff and often sore?		Do you have any food allergies?	
Do you have frequent headaches?		Do you have get fevers every year or experience chills?	
Do you get sinus infections?		Do you get heartburn?	
Do you get ear infections or blockages?		Do you get hives, itchy skin, or rash?	
Do you feel frequent fatigue?		Have you experienced unexplained appetite loss or weight loss?	
Do you get cold sores?		Do you have foul-smelling stools?	
Do you experience palpitations, panic attacks, or anxiety?		Do you have rectal bleeding?	
Have you lost hair in your eyebrows?		Do you feel depressed or irritable?	
		Do you tend to vomit frequently?	
Has your voice changed (become hoarse)?		Do you have anemia?	
Do you get a rash on your chest?		Do you crave fried food and salt once a week?	
Do you have eczema?		Do you have smelly breath in the morning?	
Have you experienced any changes in your hair (texture, falling out)?		Does your stomach get bloated?	
Do you have flaky nails, ridges on the nails, or nails that break easily?		Does your stomach often make rumbling noises?	
Have you been in a car accident and had an X-ray?		Do you get gas?	
		Are you constipated?	
Do you often feel weak?		Are your bowel movements frequent and as soon as you eat (e.g., diarrhea, loose stools)?	
Are you pale?			
Are your eyes swollen and dry?			
Are you rarely hungry for breakfast?		Do you get fever, nausea, and cramps with watery diarrhea?	

Table 18. **What's Your Back Pain Type?** (continued)

TYPE A – UPPER BACK PAIN	✓	TYPE B – LOWER BACK PAIN	✓
Are you quiet in the morning? Don't like people talking to you first thing?		Have you had your colonoscopy (if you're forty-plus)?	
Does your energy pick up after coffee?		Have you been tested for lactose intolerance?	
Are you more often cold than hot?		Have you been tested for parasite-borne diseases such as giardia or amebiasis?	
Are you able to focus well? Do you have any concentration problems?		Do you have inflammatory bowel disease?	
Do you sleep more than six to eight hours daily?		Do you have ulcerative colitis or Crohn's disease?	
Are you emotionally oversensitive?		Do you get so-called traveler's diarrhea?	
Do you fear a loss of power or loss of financial well-being?		Have you recently been to Mexico, India, Peru, or Ethiopia?	
Do you fear abandonment?		Have you taken antibiotics recently?	
Are you happy with your work environment?		Do you occasionally have a loss of appetite?	
Do you feel that the people around you are negative?		Do you get pain in your coccyx?	
Are you moody? Irritable? Snappish?		Have you ever broken your coccyx (say, falling off a horse)?	
Are you able to make decisions easily?		Do you have a history of lumbar spine fusion?	
Are you able to think about your future?		Have you ever had a disc injury?	
Are you stuck in a negative state?		Do you have leg pain?	
Are you drinking or feeding your emotions?		Do you have knee pain?	
Are you underweight?		Do you have right foot or ankle pain or swelling?	
Is your energy low?		Do you have numbness in your toes?	
Are you reserved?		Have you ever broken or overstrained a little toe?	
Have you broken any bones?		Do you suffer with plantar warts (i.e., warts on the soles of your feet)?	
Do you have osteopenia or osteoporosis or a family history of either?		Do you get smelly feet?	

Table 18. **What's Your Back Pain Type?** (continued)

TYPE A – UPPER BACK PAIN	✓	TYPE B – LOWER BACK PAIN	✓
Have you ever experienced dizzy spells or vertigo (especially when moving your neck)?		Are you often thirsty?	
		Are you more often hot than cold?	
Have you felt wobbly, weak, or sick to your stomach?		Are you gaining weight?	
		Do you have a contraceptive coil?	
Have you ever experienced inner ear conditions such as the following? 　Benign paroxysmal positional 　　vertigo (BPPV) 　Crystals in the ear 　Viral vestibular neuritis 　Tinnitus (ringing in the ear, or 　　a low sound as if the radio 　　were still on) 　Ménière's disease		Do you have hemorrhoids? (Or do they develop if you drink vodka or champagne?	
		Do you have a history of serious infection (e.g., sepsis after childbirth)?	
		Do you get a swollen vagina after sex?	
		Do you get bladder infections? Cystitis?	
Do you clench or grind your teeth? Have you had root canals, fractured teeth, crowns, or chipped teeth?		Do you have a history of PCOS?	
Do you get congested sinuses?		Do you have a history of cysts, either endometrial or dermoid (i.e., containing teeth, hair, and/or fluid)?	
Do you get a bad metallic taste in your mouth?		Do you suffer from vaginal or sacral herpes?	
Do you get eye strain?		Do you get itchiness in the anal area?	
Do you feel dizziness after being around negative people?		Do you have smelly blood during your periods?	
Do you have pain in your jaw?		Are you impulsive?	
Do you get facial pain?		Do you find it hard to forgive (especially your mom or dad)?	
Do you have a frozen shoulder or reduced range of movement and pain on one side (for example, when you try to do up your bra or do a ponytail)?		Are you lacking in self-trust?	
		Are you lacking in trust in your partner?	
Have you had teeth extractions on the same side as your neck pain?		Are you lacking in self-control?	
Have you not finished with a prescribed dental treatment?		Are you sitting on old pain (i.e., are you stubborn)?	
		Do you get stuck in relationships?	

Table 18. **What's Your Back Pain Type?** (continued)

TYPE A – UPPER BACK PAIN	✓	TYPE B – LOWER BACK PAIN	✓
Do you have a gap (or more than one gap) between teeth?		Do you have toxic relationships?	
Do you have loss of teeth? Or are you missing certain back teeth entirely (i.e., they never grew in)?		Do you have unresolved childhood trauma/abuse?	
Do you have a dental bridge or implants?		Did your parents suppress your passion or not allow you to follow your dream?	
Are you on schedule with your dentist and hygienist appointments?		Is your left foot longer than your right, or vice versa?	
Do you crave oranges and vinegar?		Do you get lower back pain if you don't wear your orthotics? Have you been tested for orthotics? Are your arches flat?	
Do you crave sugar or alcohol to help with pain?			
Do you sit or stand for long hours on the job?		Do you have big bunions (perhaps like your mother or grandmother)?	
Do you sleep with two pillows?		Do you have a white bumpy rash (which may indicate thrush/candida)?	
Do you have allergies? Hay fever?			
Do you wake up in the middle of the night angry, with anxiety, or thinking of negative things?		**TOTAL**	
Do you have yellow skin under your big toe?			
TOTAL			

The Positive Feedback Resources

With a bit of creative sleuthing, you'll soon realize you are blessed with abundant resources, both online and in stores, to support you as you adopt the Positive Feedback program. I've listed some of my favorite sources of foods and products below. If you look around, you'll also find great local suppliers specific to your town or region.

Grocery co-ops are a great place to start, whether you're looking for organic foods or organic products. If you have a co-op in your area, I heartily recommend joining it. My local co-op, called Co-opportunity, is amazing—low prices and very fresh produce, with many healthy organic brands: http://www.coopportunity.com/.

To find a co-op near you, check out this no-frills co-op directory service: http://www.coopdirectory.org/. Alternatively, check out the National Cooperative Grocers Association website: https://www.ncga.coop/.

If you don't have a co-op near you, how about starting one? Plenty of people have. If you're working toward your radiant goal and you care deeply about sustainable healthy food and workers' rights, learn more at the Cooperative Grocer website: http://www.cgin.coop/home.

Now for some specific foods and products:

Meat and Seafood

Whole Foods

By far the best national retailer for organic, free-range poultry is Whole Foods. My family and I love their yummy, fresh (not frozen) chicken.

http://www.wholefoodsmarket.com/department/article/chicken

At Whole Foods, the meat department has a clock on the display that tells you when the meat was ground. Their beef is high in quality, low in fat content, grass-fed, and raised without antibiotics.

http://www.wholefoodsmarket.com/department/article/beef

Whole Foods also has a great fish calendar (indicating which fish are freshest), as well as a calendar for fresh produce. The staff is honest when you ask for help. I always ask things like, "Can you tell me what's the best meat for two-year-olds? Can you suggest something wild, organic, and with no antibiotics or preservatives?" They do carry some farmed seafood, but I learned their farmed salmon aren't given chemical feed to enhance their color—instead, their feed includes shrimp shells to get their pink color (just like flamingos!).

http://www.wholefoodsmarket.com/department/seafood

Monterey Bay Aquarium Seafood Watch

The good people at the Monterey Bay Aquarium have a number of tools that consumers can use to make educated choices for their seafood. They have tons of information about ethical fishing practices, environmental concerns, and heavy metal toxicity, among other issues. Download their app or read more information at their website. They even have a guide to restaurants and stores (including Whole Foods!) that follow their guidelines for seafood.

**http://www.montereybayaquarium.org/cr/cr_seafoodwatch/sfw
_consumers.aspx**

Dairy Products and Processed Meats

Redwood Hill Farm Goat Yogurt

This is a delicious natural product. Add some almonds or walnuts for extra protein, and some blueberries—all of which are anti-inflammatory foods. I love to add a big spoonful of Redwood Hill Farm yogurt to my morning smoothie.

http://www.redwoodhill.com/goat-yogurt

Go Greek Yogurt

I'd like to put in a plug for my favorite smoothie connection, Go Greek, on North Bedford Drive in Beverly Hills. The owners are wonderful, and they create the most amazing yogurt blends with their own triple-strained Greek yogurt. If you're ever in Los Angeles, you owe it to yourself to check them out. I hope that they will soon branch out across the world!

http://gogreekyogurt.com

365 Everyday Value Mild Goat Cheese Slices

I use these slices on toast or for free-range cheeseburgers. So convenient and satisfying.

http://www.wholefoodsmarket.com/department/article/goat-cheese

Applegate Deli Meats

I tried several brands of roast turkey at Whole Foods, and Applegate organic was the best. It's not dry and not smoked. It has delicious flavor but contains no antibiotics, no preservatives, no nitrates—it's as natural as you can get. It's great with sliced avocados on toasted wheat-free rye bread with a drop of olive oil and a little mustard; add salad and you have a great meal. Kids love it, too.

http://www.applegate.com/products/wall-deli/category

Nondairy Milks

365 Organic Almond Milk, Unsweetened

Many almond milks are packed with sugar. I love that Whole Foods has an organic, unsweetened version. So simple and good for you, and less expensive than many of the "fancy" sugar-packed brands.

http://www.wholefoodsmarket.com/products/organic-almond milk-unsweetened

Rice Dream Vanilla Enriched Rice Drink

Rice milk is less nutritious than almond milk, but still a good alternative to dairy milk.

http://www.tastethedream.com/products/product/1474/202.php

Smoothie Mixes

Warrior Blend Classic Raw Vegan Protein Powder

My favorite is their Vanilla powder.

http://www.sunwarrior.com/product-info/warrior-blend

TerrAmazon

I've had great success with their maca, acai, cacao, and camu camu powders.

http://www.terramazon.com/eng

LivingFuel SuperBerry Ultimate

SuperBerry Ultimate is a whole-meal superfood smoothie mix that combines concentrated superfoods and nutrients from high-quality organic, all-natural sources. The LivingFuel company recommends that you start with this product (as opposed to the next one listed), as its milder flavor appeals to both adults and kids.

http://www.livingfuel.com/Living-Fuel-Rx-Super-Berry-Ultimate.aspx

LivingFuel SuperGreens

SuperGreens has an almost two-to-one protein-to-carbohydrate ratio and a two-to-one carbohydrate-to-fiber ratio. Therefore, you can mix in small amounts of any kind of juice or fruit and still not raise your blood sugar level significantly. This mix is full of organic veggies and grasses—barley, broccoli, spinach, kale, carrots, spirulina, and more.

http://www.livingfuel.com/Living-Fuel-Rx-Super-Greens.aspx

Jay Robb Egg White Protein Powder

This non-GMO powder comes in vanilla, chocolate, strawberry, and unflavored. I love that it has 24 grams of protein and no sugar.

http://www.jayrobb.com/protein/egg-white-protein-vanilla.asp

Grains

Lundberg Short-Grain Organic Brown Rice

This rice is so nutty and flavorful that I add just olive oil, lemon, and sea salt.

**http://www.lundberg.com/products/rice/packaged_rice/Short_Grain
_Brown_Organic.aspx**

Bob's Red Mill Organic Rolled Oats

I eat some variety of Bob's Red Mill Oats almost every morning— I love all of their products.

http://www.bobsredmill.com/organic-regular-rolled-oats.html

Pastas

Ancient Harvest Quinoa Supergrain Pasta

The manufacturer's slogan for this gluten-free product is "You'll never go back to 'plain' noodles again!"—and I so agree. This is my favorite spaghetti!

http://store.ancientharvestquinoa.com/Organic-Quinoa-Pastas/c/ AncientHarvest@Pasta

Andean Dream Quinoa Pasta

These gluten- and corn-free organic noodles are yummy.

http://www.andeandream.com/OtherProducts.html

VitaSpelt Organic Spelt Pasta

This is another delicious, wholesome pasta. Spelt is known as "zea" wheat in Greece, and it's much more common in Europe. The original strain of wheat that's existed for nine thousand years before modern hybridization, spelt has less reactive gluten and is easier to digest than other kinds of wheat.

https://www.natureslegacyforlife.com/shopping/pastas

Tinkyada Pasta Joy Organic Brown Rice Pasta

Many prefer the taste of rice pasta. This kind is made entirely of brown rice and has more nutrients and fiber than white rice pasta.

http://www.tinkyada.com/

Breads

Mestemacher Natural Whole Rye
Bread (with whole rye kernels)

This yummy rye is great toasted with a little olive oil, or with thin slices of Applegate roast turkey and a little lettuce or mustard.

http://www.mestemacher-gmbh.com/product-line/organic-breads/
natural-whole-rye-bread

Food for Life Ezekiel 4:9 Bread

Available in almost every decent grocery store, this bread is packed with nutrition and palatable for all family members.

http://www.foodforlife.com/about_us/ezekiel-49

Pancake Mix

Namaste Waffle and Pancake Mix

This gluten-free mix isn't organic, but it is GMO-free and has no preservatives. Its ingredients include brown rice, tapioca, and arrowroot flours. To make it in the most health-supportive way, use rice or almond milk, organic eggs, and olive oil or coconut oil.

http://www.namastefoods.com/products/cgi-bin/products
.cgi?Function=show&Id=23

Arrowhead Mills Organic Gluten-Free
Pancake and Baking Mix

Add your own almond milk, organic eggs, and coconut oil to make this delicious treat.

http://www.arrowheadmills.com/product/organic-gluten-free-pancake
-and-baking-mix

Cereal

Nature's Path Organic Millet Rice Cereal with Oatbran

Eaten with almond milk, this cereal is crunchy and delicious.

http://shop.naturespath.com/Millet-Rice-Flakes/p/NPA

-770077&c=NaturesPath@ColdCereals

Oatmeal and Yogurt Toppings

Himalania Goji Berries

I put these in everything—oatmeal, yogurt, salads, smoothies! Goji berries have tons of antioxidants, vitamin C, fiber, iron, and other nutrients that improve circulation, immunity, endurance, and stamina.

http://www.brandstorminc.com/gojiberries.php

Himalania Hemp Seeds/Chia Seeds

Both these types of seeds add extra nutrition, including amino acids, fiber, omega-3s, protein—and a nice crunch!—to oatmeal and yogurt. (I sometimes throw them into smoothies and soup, too.)

http://www.brandstorminc.com/hempseeds.php,

http://www.brandstorminc.com/chiaseeds.php

TerrAmazon Raw Organic Cacao Nibs

I sprinkle these over yogurt, mix them with nuts, or just eat a couple for a quick lift.

http://www.terramazon.com/eng

Nut and Seed Butters and Oils

Artisana Organic Almond Butter
This is a good source of protein. Spread on rye wheat-free bread with honey, banana, and some goji berries, it makes a delicious dessert. Great as a snack for kids, also.
http://www.Artisans foods.com

MaraNatha Organic Raw Almond Butter
You can't get healthier than this. I love this almond butter in my oatmeal in the morning.
http://www.maranathafoods.com/category/almond-butters/organic

Living Tree Community Foods Almond
Butter and Sesame Tahini
I love these two nut butters on Ezekiel bread with banana.
http://www.livingtreecommunity.com

Nutiva Organic Extra-Virgin Coconut Oil
I love everything about this product, from eating it to smelling it to using it on my skin! I use it to massage patients. It's even great on hair! In addition, coconut oil has antifungal, antiviral, and anti-bacterial properties. For example, it kills yeast infections in the intestine and reduces inflammation and gut problems that can cause lower back pain and other problems.
http://nutiva.com/products/coconut-oil-organic-benefits-nutiva

Snacks

Alive & Radiant Foods Organic Kale Krunch

These spicy kale chips are great for on-the-go snacking.

http://shop.kaiafoods.com

Blue Diamond Nut Thins (Almond Flavor)

These crackers are made with almonds and nuts—crunchy and gluten-free. Also available in pecan.

http://bluediamond.com/index.cfm?navid=54

Keen-Wäh Decadence Protein Bars

Treat yourself while gaining valuable protein—yummy!

http://www.keenwah.com

Hail Merry Macaroons

Available in a range of flavors, these gluten-free vegan treats contain raw oils and no refined sugar.

http://www.hailmerry.com/macaroons

Nature's All Freeze-Dried Bananas

This company's organic, fair-trade-certified products (many fruits available) are vegan and gluten-free.

http://www.naturesallfoods.com

Vegetable Stock

Rapunzel Vegan Vegetable Bouillon with Sea Salt

This delicious vegetable stock is great in any recipe calling for stock.

http://www.rapunzel.de/uk/p_wuerzmittel.html

Salts

Himalania Himalayan Pink Salt

This salt is delicious and has over eighty-four naturally rich elements and trace minerals such as iron, magnesium, calcium, chromium, copper, and zinc.

http://www.brandstorminc.com/pinksalt.php

Teas and Other Beverages

Greek Mountain Tea (Mt. Taygetos)

This Greek whole-leaf tea is marvelously relaxing and useful in fending off colds and flu during the winter.

http://www.greekinternetmarket.com/1050-03001.html

Traditional Medicinals Organic Nettle Leaf Tea

I love this anti-inflammatory tea—I drink it all day long. Nettle is a very particular taste, though. Start with one cup a day or alternate it with other teas. (All of Traditional Medicinals Teas are very high quality.)

http://www.traditionalmedicinals.com/product/nettle-leaf

American Tea Room

Many of their teas are so delicious, you can substitute them for any dessert! I especially like the Choco*Late Organic Tea (a caffeine-free hot chocolate alternative), the Brioche Organic Tea (tastes like a pastry), and the Oriental Beauty Oolong Tea (although not organic, the maple and walnut flavors are delicious).

http://www.americantearoom.com

Synergy Kombucha
My favorite flavor is Cherry Chia, but I love all of them.
http://synergydrinks.com

Organic Avenue Boosters
These are only available in New York right now, but they're perfect for when I'm there on business and feeling a little extra stress. I especially love the Lemon Shot.
http://www.organicavenue.com/juices/booster-shots.html

Pressed Juicery
These juice cleanses and cold-pressed juices are some of the most delicious I've ever tasted! You can either visit one of their locations in California or have them shipped right to your door.
http://www.pressedjuicery.com/

Vitamins and Supplements

New Chapter Vitamins
I love several of this company's formulations: Every Woman, Activated C Food Complex and Wholemega Whole Fish Oil.
http://www.newchapter.com/vitamins

California Natural Immunity Shots
This formula contains ginger and colloidal silver, oregano oil, grapefruit seed extract, and zinc. It keeps me healthy when I travel.
https://www.californianatural.net/products_Detail.php?ProductID=9

Barlean's Olive Leaf Complex Throat Spray
I recommend this spray to all of my singing or acting clients, to keep their throats healthy, especially during the winter months.
http://www.barleans.com/literature/olc-spray.pdf

Sovereign Silver

This colloidal silver product is useful for its antibacterial and antifungal properties. The spray helps bolster the immune system, especially when you're going into an area with lots of germs (e.g., on a plane or in another public, enclosed space). Some people also use topical colloidal silver to help with burns, acne, and other skin irritations.

http://www.natural-immunogenics.com

Udo's Choice Ultimate Oil Blend

This organic seed oil blend mixes essential fatty acids Omega 3, alpha linolenic acid (ALA), and linoleic acid (LA) together with the fatty acid Omega 9 in a 2:1:1 ratio. Udo's Choice is made in the UK, but you can get it on Amazon.com in the United States.

http://www.udoschoice.co.uk/products/udos-choice-ultimate-oil
-blend#sthash.I563Vqsy.dpuf

Natural Factors Oil of Oregano

Oil of oregano is a versatile antibacterial, antifungal, and antiparasitic remedy that I recommend to everyone who travels often or encounters a lot of immune system challenges from other people's germs (public transport, crowded offices, working in public health settings, and so on).

http://naturalfactors.com/Frontend/WebsiteImages/naturalfactorscanada/
documents/874__Oregano-RS.pdf.pdf

Comvita Propolis Oral Spray

This spray, with manuka honey, boasts antibacterial qualities and can help soothe sore throats. (Please steer clear if you are allergic to bee stings.)

http://www.comvita.com/healthcare/propolis/propolis-oral-spray.html

OLLOÏS Homeopathic Medicine

Their homeopathic medicines are made in France from high-quality ingredients and no synthetic chemicals.

http://www.ollois.com

Dry Brushes

Bass Body Care

This company carries brushes, loofahs, and scrubbing mitts. If you can't find a brush, you can use a loofah. Bass Body Care loofahs work well dry. Many people prefer to use them wet, however, followed by a visit to a steam room to sweat (and then, if possible, a jump into cold water).

http://www.amazon.com/Vegetable-Bristle-Skin-Body-Brush/dp/B000HCNHSI

Sublime Beauty Body Brush

This brush seems to be the right texture for dry brushing, with many positive user reviews on Amazon. (In truth, any natural bristle body brush should work, so just look for one in your price range and your desired style [long handled or short].)

http://sublime-beauty.net/skinbrushing

Exercise Plans and Tools

Jawbone UP

This wristband and app track what you eat, how you move, and how much and how deeply you sleep. You can share your information with friends, a feature I love to use with my patients: I can track their progress and send them motivating and congratulatory messages from the road. My friends and I have become hooked on this device!

https://jawbone.com/up

Tracy Anderson Method

Many of my patients swear by Tracy Anderson Method. Her approach is different in that it challenges small muscle groups with resistance and forces your body to rely on your own balance. This approach strengthens the smaller muscle groups so that these muscles can pull in the larger muscles—which results in a lean figure that is not bulky.

http://tracyandersonmethod.com

Osteopaths and Naturopaths

American Osteopathic Association

In the States, osteopathic physicians, or DOs, practice a "whole-person" approach to health care and receive special training in the musculoskeletal system. In contrast to European Osteopaths, DOs can prescribe pharmaceuticals, do surgery, and have training and credentials similar to those of an MD.

http://www.osteopathic.org

International Osteopathic Association

In contrast to American osteopathy, European osteopathy focuses on disorders of the neuromusculoskeletal and joint system, and the effects of these disorders on general health, practicing a drug-free, hands-on approach to health care. In addition to manual therapy, European osteopaths are also trained to recommend therapeutic and rehabilitative exercises, as well as to provide nutritional, dietary, and lifestyle counseling and administer physiological therapeutic modalities (such as acupuncture, cranial sacral therapy, spinal and deep tissue manipulation, etc.).

http://www.internationalosteopathicassociation.org

American Association of Naturopathic Physicians

For patients in the States who are interested in but do not have access to European osteopaths, naturopathic doctors may be a good choice as they bridge some abilities of both US and European style osteopaths. Naturopathic practice includes the following diagnostic and therapeutic modalities: clinical and laboratory diagnostic testing, nutritional medicine, botanical medicine, naturopathic physical medicine (including naturopathic manipulative therapy), public health measures, hygiene, counseling, homeopathy, acupuncture, prescription medication, and naturopathic obstetrics (natural childbirth).

http://www.naturopathic.org

EMDR Practitioners

EMDR International Association

More and more therapists and psychologists are becoming trained in EMDR every day. Seek out a licensed practitioner in your area.

http://www.emdria.org

The Positive Feedback Shopping List

Sample Shopping List for Release

The Positive Feedback Meal Plan is customizable to your personal tastes. I'll give you a sample shopping list that you can take with you for the first week. (Note: Please use this shopping list as a guide, not a mandate. Everyone has different tastes, family members, budgets, available food items. I offer this as a general guideline more than a prescription. Please make your choices according to what is in season, in your budget, and to your preference.

Most of my patients find that they reconnect with their food and start to enjoy their shopping and cooking experiences much more and they begin to develop their own approaches that are based on the Positive Feedback principles. For example, the smoothie recipes are truly infinitely adjustable—you will definitely begin to develop favorite combinations and ratios of ingredients, which is wonderful.

If you're a bit out of touch with your local grocer or farmer's market, you can use this list as a starting point. But I encourage you to develop your own lists in the subsequent weeks—I want you to own food shopping as an intricate piece of Positive Feedback way of life.

Produce

   1 bag of baby spinach
   1 bag of other lettuce (romaine, spring mix, etc.)
   1 bag or bunch of other green leafy vegetables
   1 avocado
   3 large red peppers
   3 large grapefruits (1 for each day of the Liver Cleanse)
   1 large bag of lemons
   1 pumpkin
   1 squash (variety to taste)
   3 sweet potatoes
   1 zucchini
   1 pomegranate (or container of pomegranate seeds)
   1 small piece of fresh ginger
   1 bunch of broccoli
   1 bunch of asparagus
   7 onions (combination of yellow and white—1 per day)
   1 bunch cilantro or 1 bunch parsley
   1 bunch fresh carrots
   1 head of celery
   1 bunch vine-ripened tomatoes
   1 bulb of garlic
   3 bananas
   1 to 2 packages of berries (blueberries, raspberries, or blackberries)
   2 peaches or mangoes
   2 kiwi

Packaged Goods

   1 container of sea salt
   1 container of peppercorns for grinding
   1 container of steel-cut rolled oats

2 bags of dried beans (alfalfa, mung, black-eyed peas, or similar)

1 package of walnuts

1 package of pecans

1 package of almonds

1 package of raw cashews

1 package of pine nuts (optional)

1 package of pumpkin seeds

1 package of goji berries

1 package of sunflower seeds

1 small jar of almond butter

1 large bottle of extra-virgin olive oil (the best quality you can afford)

1 or 2 packages of tea (fennel, nettle, peppermint leaf, anise, green, jasmine)

1 container of smoothie protein powder

Cold Items

1 container of coconut water (optional)

1 dozen eggs

1 package of vegetable bouillon cubes

1 package of crumbled feta (goat's or sheep's milk)

½ gallon unsweetened almond milk

1 container of plain goat's milk yogurt

2 to 3 pieces of fish (for latter half of week)

2 to 3 slices of fresh pineapple (or whole pineapple from produce aisle)

Notes

Introduction

1. Ethan K., M. G. Berman, W. Mischel, and others, "Social Rejection Shares Somatosensory Representations with Physical Pain," *Proceedings of the National Academy of Sciences* 108, no. 15 (2011): 6270–6275; Epub: Mar. 28, 2011, doi:10.1073/pnas.1102693108.

2. H. R. Eriksen, H. Ursin, "Subjective Health Complaints, Sensitization, and Sustained Cognitive Activation (Stress)," *Journal of Psychosomatic Research* 56, no. 4 (Apr. 2004): 445–48. Review. PubMed PMID: 15094030.

Chapter 1. What Is Pain?

1. J. F. Brosschot, W. Gerin, and J. F. Thayer, "The Perseverative Cognition Hypothesis: A Review of Worry, Prolonged Stress-Related Physiological Activation, and Health," *Journal of Psychosomatic Research* 60, no. 2 (Feb. 2006): 113–24. Review. PubMed PMID: 16439263.

2. P. T. Dorsher, "Can Classical Acupuncture Points and Trigger Points Be Compared in the Treatment of Pain Disorders? Birch's Analysis Revisited," *Journal of Alternative and Complementary Medicine* 14, no. 4 (May 2008): 353–59, doi:10.1089/acm.2007.0810. Review. PubMed PMID: 18576919.

3. B. Verkuil, J. F. Brosschot, W. A. Gebhardt, and J. F. Thayer, "When Worries Make You Sick: A Review of Perseverative Cognition, the Default Stress Response and Somatic Health," *Journal of Experimental Psychopathology* 1, no. 1 (2010): 87–118, doi:10.5127/jep.009110.

4. R. Martone, "Scientists Discover Children's Cells Living in Mothers' Brains," *Scientific American,* Dec. 4, 2012 (http://www.scientificamerican.com/article.cfm?id=scientists-discover-childrens-cells-living-in-mothers-brain).

5. J. L. St. Sauver, D. O. Warner, B. P. Yawn, and others, "Why Patients Visit Their Doctors: Assessing the Most Prevalent Conditions in a Defined American Population," *Mayo Clinic Proceedings* 88, no. 1 (Jan. 2013): 56–67, doi:10.1016/j.mayocp.2012.08.020.

6. S. Glover and L. Girion, "Deaths Tied to Painkillers Rising in the U.S.," *Los Angeles Times,* Mar. 29, 2013 (http://www.latimes.com/news/local/la-me-0330-rx-deaths-20130330,0,1604889.story).

7. A. Zuger, "Hard Cases: The Traps of Treating Pain," *New York Times,* May 13, 2013 (http://well.blogs.nytimes.com/2013/05/13/hard-cases-the-traps-of-treating-pain).

8. S. Tavernise, "Sharp Rise in Women's Deaths from Overdose of Painkillers," *New York Times,* July 2, 2013 (http://www.nytimes.com/2013/07/03/health/rate-of-painkiller -overdose-deaths-rises-among-women.html).

9. Centers for Disease Control and Prevention, "Prescription Painkiller Overdoses," *CDC Vital Signs,* July 2013. (http://www.cdc.gov/vitalsigns/PrescriptionPainkillerOverdoses/ index.html).

10. Centers for Disease Control and Prevention. "Prescription Painkiller Overdoses," *CDC Vital Signs,* July 2013 (http://www.cdc.gov/vitalsigns/PrescriptionPainkillerOverdoses/ index.html).

11. Centers for Disease Control and Prevention. "Prescription Painkiller Overdoses," *CDC Vital Signs,* July 2013 (http://www.cdc.gov/vitalsigns/PrescriptionPainkillerOverdoses/ index.html).

12. Centers for Disease Control and Prevention. "Prescription Painkiller Overdoses," *CDC Vital Signs,* July 2013 (http://www.cdc.gov/vitalsigns/PrescriptionPainkillerOverdoses/ index.html).

13. Caroline Stone, *Science in the Art of Osteopathy: Osteopathic Principles and Practice* (Cheltenham: Nelson Thornes, Ltd., 2002), 82.

14. R. Hanson, "Relaxed and Contented: Activating the Parasympathetic Wing of Your Nervous System," http://www.wisebrain.org/ParasympatheticNS.pdf.

15. P. Gilbert, "Introducing Compassion-focused Therapy," *Advances in Psychiatric Treatment* 15 (2009): 199–208, doi:10 1192/apt.bp.107.005264.

16. A. van Santen, S. A. Vreeburg, A. J. Van der Does, and others, "Psychological Traits and the Cortisol Awakening Response: Results from the Netherlands Study of Depression and Anxiety," *Psychoneuroendocrinology* 36, no. 2 (Feb. 2011): 240–48, doi:10.1016/j. psyneuen.2010.07.014. Epub 2010 Aug 17. PubMed PMID: 20724080.

17. R. Hanson, "Relaxed and Contented: Activating the Parasympathetic Wing of Your Nervous System," http://www.wisebrain.org/ParasympatheticNS.pdf.

18. M. A. Fischer, "Manic Nation: Dr. Peter Whybrow Says We're Addicted to Stress," *Pacific Standard,* June 19, 2012 (http://www.psmag.com/health/manic-nation-dr-peter -whybrow-says-were-addicted-stress-42695/).

19. S. Cohen, N. Hamrick, M. S. Rodriguez, and others, "Reactivity and Vulnerability to Stress-Associated Risk for Upper Respiratory Illness," *Psychosomatic Medicine* 64, no. 2 (Mar./Apr. 2002): 302–10. PubMed PMID: 11914447.

20. R. F. Baumeister, E. Bratslavsky, C. Finkenauer, and K. D. Vohs, "Bad Is Stronger Than Good," *Review of General Psychology* 5, no. 4 (2001): 323–70 1089–2680/O1/S5.OO doi:10.1037//1089–2680.5.4.323.

21. P. Rozin and E. B. Royzman, "Negativity Bias, Negativity Dominance, and Contagion," *Personality and Social Psychology Review* 5 (Nov. 2001): 296–320, doi:10.1207/ S15327957PSPR0504_2.

22. P. Pervanidou and G. P. Chrousos, "Metabolic Consequences of Stress During Childhood and Adolescence," *Metabolism* 61, no. 5 (May 2012): 611–19, doi:10.1016/j .metabol.2011.10.005; P. Pervanidou and G. P. Chrousos, "Posttraumatic Stress Disorder in Children and Adolescents: Neuroendocrine Perspectives," *Science Signaling* 9, no. 5 (Oct. 2012): 245, doi:10.1126/scisignal.2003327. PubMed PMID: 23047921.

23. R. Hanson, "Relaxed and Contented: Activating the Parasympathetic Wing of Your Nervous System," http://www.wisebrain.org/ParasympatheticNS.pdf.

24. T. Pramanik, H.O. Sharma, S. Mishra, and others, "Immediate Effect of Slow Pace Bhastrika Pranayama on Blood Pressure and Heart Rate," *Journal of Alternative and Complementary Medicine* 15, no. 3 (Mar. 2009): 293–95.

25. M. Rosengård-Bärlund, L. Bernardi, A. Sandelin, and others, "Baroreflex Sensitivity and Its Response to Deep Breathing Predict Increase in Blood Pressure in Type 1 Diabetes in a 5-Year Follow-up," *Diabetes Care* 34, no. 11 (Nov. 2011): 2424–30.

26. N. Moore, D. Brown, N. Money, and M. Bates, "Mind Body Skills for Regulating the Autonomic Nervous System," Defense Centers of Excellence for Psychological Health and Traumatic Brain Injury, v. 2 (July 2011) (http://www.dcoe.mil/Content/Navigation/Documents/Mind-Body%20Skills%20for%20Regulating%20the%20Autonomic%20Nervous%20System.pdf)

Chapter 2. Living in the Positive

1. C. E. Kerr, M. D. Sacchet, S. W. Lazar, C. I. Moore, and S. R. Jones, "Mindfulness Starts with the Body: Somatosensory Attention and Top-Down Modulation of Cortical Alpha Rhythms in Mindfulness Meditation," *Frontiers in Human Neuroscience* 7, no. 12. (2013), doi: 10.3389/fnhum.2013.00012.

Chapter 3. How the Positive Feedback Program Works

1. C. E. Kerr, M. D. Sacchet, S. W. Lazar, and others, "Mindfulness Starts with the Body: Somatosensory Attention and Top-Down Modulation of Cortical Alpha Rhythms in Mindfulness Meditation," *Frontiers in Human Neuroscience* 7, no. 12. (2013), doi:10.3389/fnhum.2013.00012.

2. F. Zeidan, K. T. Martucci, R. A. Kraft, and others, "Brain Mechanisms Supporting the Modulation of Pain by Mindfulness Meditation," *Journal of Neuroscience* 31, no. 14 (Apr. 6, 2011): 5540–48, doi:10.1523/JNEUROSCI.5791-10.2011.PubMed PMID: 21471390; PubMed Central PMCID: PMC3090218.

3. "Sugar-Sweetened Beverages, Obesity, and Chronic Disease Fact Sheet," Boston Public Health Commission (http://www.bphc.org/programs/cib/chronicdisease/sugarsmarts/aboutthecampaign/Documents/SugarSweetenedBeverageFactSheet.pdf).

4. B. K. Hölzel, J. Carmody, M. Vangel, and others, "Mindfulness Practice Leads to Increases in Regional Brain Gray Matter Density," *Psychiatry Research* 191, no. 1 (Jan. 30, 2011): 36–43, doi:10.1016/j.pscychresns.2010.08.006. Epub 2010 Nov 10. PubMed PMID: 21071182; PubMed Central PMCID: PMC3004979.

5. R. Sapolsky, "Stress and Your Shrinking Brain," *Discover* 20, no. 3 (1999): 116–22.

6. W. Hofmann, M. Luhmann, R. R. Fisher, and others, "Yes, But Are They Happy? Effects of Trait Self-Control on Affective Well-Being and Life Satisfaction," *Journal of Personality* (June 11, 2013), doi:10.1111/jopy.12050. [Epub ahead of print] PubMed PMID: 23750741.

7. E. Golden, A. Emiliano, S. Maudsley, and others, "Circulating Brain-Derived Neurotrophic Factor and Indices of Metabolic and Cardiovascular Health: Data from the Baltimore Longitudinal Study of Aging." *PLoS ONE* 5, no. 4 (2010): e10099, doi:10.1371/journal.pone.0010099; S. M. Rothman, K. J. Griffioen, R. Wan, M. P. Mattson, "Brain-derived Neurotrophic Factor as a Regulator of Systemic and Brain Energy Metabolism and Cardiovascular Health," *Annals of the New York Academy of Sciences* 1264, no. 1 (Aug. 2012):49–63, doi:10.1111/j.1749-6632.2012.06525.x. Epub 2012 Apr 30. Review. PubMed PMID: 22548651; PubMed Central PMCID: PMC3411899.

8. P. Condon, G. Desbordes, W. B. Miller, D. Desteno, "Meditation Increases Compassionate Responses to Suffering," Psychological Science 24, no. 10 (Oct. 1, 2013): 2125–27, doi:10.1177/0956797613485603. Epub 2013 Aug 21. PubMed PMID: 23965376.

9. S. Jeffers, *Feel the Fear and Do it Anyway* (New York, Random House: 1987).

Chapter 4. Week 1: Reflect

1. K. Minoguchi, T. Tazaki, and T. Yokoe, "Elevated Production of Tumor Necrosis Factor-α by Monocytes in Patients with Obstructive Sleep Apnea Syndrome," *Chest* 126 (2004): 1473–79.

2. L. Xie, H. Kang, Q. Xu, and others, "Sleep Drives Metabolite Clearance from the Adult Brain," *Science* 342, no. 6156 (Oct. 18, 2013): 373–37, doi:10.1126/science.1241224. PubMed PMID: 24136970; J. J. Iliff, M. Wang, Y. Liao, and others, "A Paravascular Pathway Facilitates CSF Flow Through the Brain Parenchyma and the Clearance of Interstitial Solutes, Including Amyloid β," *Science Translational Medicine* (2012), doi:10.1126/scitranslmed.3003748.

3. N. Carmen, "The Power of Rituals in Life, Death, and Business," *Harvard Business School Working Knowledge,* June 2, 2013.

4. A. E. Bonomi, M. L. Anderson, J. Nemeth, and others, "Dating Violence Victimization Across the Teen Years: Abuse Frequency, Number of Abusive Partners, and Age at First Occurrence," *BMC Public Health* 12 (Aug. 10, 2012): 637, doi:10.1186/1471-2458-12-637. PubMed PMID: 22882898; PubMed Central PMCID: PMC3490892.

5. M. L. Loureiro, S. T. Yen, and R. M. Nayga Jr. "The Effects of Nutritional Labels on Obesity." *Agricultural Economics* 43, no. 3 (2012): 333, doi:10.1111/j.1574-0862.2012.00586.x.

6. J. Dalen, B. W. Smith, B. M. Shelley, and others, "Pilot Study: Mindful Eating and Living (MEAL): Weight, Eating Behavior, and Psychological Outcomes Associated with a Mindfulness-Based Intervention for People with Obesity," *Complementary Therapies in Medicine* 18, no. 6 (Dec. 2010): 260–64, doi:10.1016/j.ctim.2010.09.008.

7. C. K. Miller, J. L. Kristeller, A. Headings, and others, "Comparative Effectiveness of a Mindful Eating Intervention to a Diabetes Self-Management Intervention Among Adults with Type 2 Diabetes: A Pilot Study," *Journal of the Academy of Nutrition and Dietetics* 112, no. 11 (Nov. 2012): 1835–42, doi:10.1016/j.jand.2012.07.036.

8. R. G. Wanden-Berghe, J. Sanz-Valero, and C. Wanden-Berghe, "The Application of Mindfulness to Eating Disorders Treatment: A Systematic Review," *Eating Disorders* 19, no. 1 (Jan. 2011): 34–48, doi:10.1080/10640266.2011.533604.

9. "Simple, Daily Steps Can Reduce Risk of Heart Disease, Mayo Clinic Experts Say," http://www.mayoclinic.org/news2013-rst/7292.html.

10. S. G. Hofmann and J. A. Smits, "Cognitive-Behavioral Therapy for Adult Anxiety Disorders: A Meta-Analysis of Randomized Placebo-Controlled Trials," *Journal of Clinical Psychiatry* 69, no. 4 (Apr. 2008): 621–32.

11. O. Doehrmann, S. S. Ghosh, F. E. Polli, and others, "Predicting Treatment Response in Social Anxiety Disorder from Functional Magnetic Resonance Imaging," *JAMA Psychiatry* 70, no. 1 (Jan. 2013): 87–97, doi:10.1001/2013.jamapsychiatry.5.

12. Mayo Clinic Staff, "Meditation: A Simple, Fast Way to Reduce Stress," http://www.mayoclinic.com/health/meditation/HQ01070.

13. P. Malinowski, "Neural Mechanisms of Attentional Control in Mindfulness Meditation," *Frontiers of Neuroscience* 4, no. 7 (Feb. 2013): 8, doi:10.3389/fnins.2013.00008 . eCollection 2013. PubMed PMID: 23382709; PubMed Central PMCID: PMC3563089; S.

Chaiopanont, "Hypoglycemic Effect of Sitting Breathing Meditation Exercise on Type 2 Diabetes at Wat Khae Nok Primary Health Center in Nonthaburi Province," *Journal of the Medical Association of Thailand* 91, no. 1 (Jan. 2008): 93–98. PubMed PMID: 18386551; D. Martarelli, M. Cocchioni, S. Scuri, and P. Pompei, "Diaphragmatic Breathing Reduces Postprandial Oxidative Stress," *Journal of Alternative and Complementary Medicine* 17, no. 7 (July 2011): 623–28, doi:10.1089/acm.2010.0666. Epub 2011 Jun 20. PubMed PMID: 21688985.

14.   E. Epel, J. Daubenmier, J. T. Moskowitz, and others, "Can Meditation Slow Rate of Cellular Aging? Cognitive Stress, Mindfulness, and Telomeres," *Annals of New York Academy of Sciences* 1172 (Aug. 2009): 34-53, doi:10.1111/j.1749-6632.2009.04414.x. Review. PubMed PMID: 19735238; PubMed Central PMCID: PMC3057175; E. A. Hoge, M. M. Chen, E. Orr, and others, "Loving-Kindness Meditation Practice Associated with Longer Telomeres in Women," *Brain, Behavior, and Immunity* 32 (Aug. 2013): 159–63, doi:10.1016/j.bbi.2013.04.005. Epub 2013 Apr 19. PubMed PMID: 23602876.

15.   H. Lavretsky, E. S. Epel, P. Siddarth, and others, "A Pilot Study of Yogic Meditation for Family Dementia Caregivers with Depressive Symptoms: Effects on Mental Health, Cognition, and Telomerase Activity." *International Journal of Geriatric Psychiatry* 28, no.1 (Jan. 2012): 57–65, doi:10.1002/gps.3790. Epub 2012 Mar 11. PubMed PMID: 22407663; PubMed Central PMCID: PMC3423469.

16.   National Center for Complementary and Alternative Medicine, "Meditation: An Introduction," http://nccam.nih.gov/health/meditation/overview.htm.

17.   F. Zeidan, K. T. Martucci, R. A. Kraft, and others, "Brain Mechanisms Supporting the Modulation of Pain by Mindfulness Meditation," *Journal of Neuroscience* 31, no. 14 (Apr. 2011): 5540–48, doi:10.1523/jneurosci.5791-10.2011.

Chapter 5. Week 2: Release

1.   A. O'Donovan, A. J. Tomiyama, J. Lin, and others, "Stress Appraisals and Cellular Aging: A Key Role for Anticipatory Threat in the Relationship Between Psychological Stress and Telomere Length," *Brain, Behavior, and Immunity* 26, no. 4 (May 2012): 573–79, doi:10.1016/j.bbi.2012.01.007.

2.   B. Berkowsky, "Skin Brushing: Rejuvenation, Circulation, and Vital Chi," *Massage & Bodywork* (Oct./Nov. 2000).

3.   R. Jerath, J. W. Edry, V. A. Barnes, and V. Jerath, "Physiology of Long Pranayamic Breathing: Neural Respiratory Elements May Provide a Mechanism That Explains How Slow Deep Breathing Shifts the Autonomic Nervous System," *Medical Hypotheses* 67, no. 3 (2006): 566–71.

4.   S. W. S. Lee and N. Schwarz, "Wiping the Slate Clean: Psychological Consequences of Physical Cleansing," *Current Directions in Psychological Science* 20 (Oct. 2011): 307–11, doi:10.1177/0963721411422694.

5.   A. Sánchez-Villegas, L. Verberne, J. De Irala, and others, "Dietary Fat Intake and the Risk of Depression: The SUN Project," *PLoS One* 6, no. 1 (Jan. 26, 2011): e16268, doi:10.1371/journal.pone.0016268. PubMed PMID: 21298116; PubMed Central PMCID:PMC3027671.

6.   B. A. Golomb, M. A. Evans, H. L. White, and J. E. Dimsdale, "Trans Fat Consumption and Aggression," *PLoS One* 7, no. 3 (2012): e32175, doi:10.1371/journal.pone.0032175. Epub 2012 Mar 5. PubMed PMID: 22403632; PubMed Central PMCID: PMC3293881.

7.   D. Estadella, C. M. da Penha Oller do Nascimento, L. M. Oyama, and others, "Lipotoxicity: Effects of Dietary Saturated and Transfatty Acids," *Mediators of Inflammation*

(2013): 137579, doi:10.1155/2013/137579. Epub 2013 Jan 31. PubMed PMID: 23509418; PubMed Central PMCID: PMC3572653.

   8.   M. P. Mattson and A. Cheng, "Neurohormetic Phytochemicals: Low-Dose Toxins That Induce Adaptive Neuronal Stress Responses," *Trends in Neuroscience* 29, no. 11 (Nov. 2006): 632–39. Epub 2006 Sep 26. Review. PubMed PMID: 17000014.

   9.   H. Arguin, I. J. Dionne, M. Sénéchal, and others, "Short- and Long-Term Effects of Continuous Versus Intermittent Restrictive Diet Approaches on Body Composition and the Metabolic Profile in Overweight and Obese Postmenopausal Women: A Pilot Study," *Menopause* 19, no. 8 (Aug. 2012): 870–76. PubMed PMID: 22735163; M. N. Harvie, M. Pegington, M. P. Mattson, and others, "The Effects of Intermittent or Continuous Energy Restriction on Weight Loss and Metabolic Disease Risk Markers: A Randomized Trial in Young Overweight Women," *International Journal of Obesity* (London) 35, no. 5 (May 2011): 714–27, doi:10.1038/ijo.2010.171. Epub 2010 Oct 5. PubMed PMID: 20921964; PubMed Central PMCID: PMC3017674.

   10.   F. R. de Azevedo, D. Ikeoka, and B. Caramelli, "Effects of Intermittent Fasting on Metabolism in Men," *Revista da Associacao Medica Brasileira* 59, no. 2 (Mar./Apr. 2013): 167–73, doi:10.1016/j.ramb.2012.09.003. PubMed PMID: 23582559.

   11.   L. Lucas, A. Russell, and R. Keast, "Molecular Mechanisms of Inflammation: Anti-Inflammatory Benefits of Virgin Olive Oil and the Phenolic Compound Oleocanthal," *Current Pharmaceutical Design* 17, no. 8 (2011): 754–68.

   12.   P. S. Larmo, A. J. Kangas, P. Soininen, and others, "Effects of Sea Buckthorn and Bilberry on Serum Metabolites Differ According to Baseline Metabolic Profiles in Overweight Women: A Randomized Crossover Trial," *American Journal of Clinical Nutrition,* Oct. 2013, 98(4): 941–51, doi:10.3945/ajcn.113.060590. Epub 2013 Aug 14. PubMed PMID: 23945716; PubMed Central PMCID: PMC3778864.

   13.   J. C. Antvorskov, P. Fundova, K. Buschard, and D. P. Funda, "Dietary Gluten Alters the Balance of Pro-Inflammatory and Anti-Inflammatory Cytokines in T Cells of BALB/C Mice," *Immunology* 138, no. 1 (Jan. 2013): 23–33, doi:10.1111/imm.12007.

   14.   Gina Kolata, "Culprit in Heart Disease Goes Beyond Meat's Fat," *New York Times,* April 7, 2013 (http://www.nytimes.com/2013/04/08/health/study-points-to-new-culprit-in -heart-disease.html).

   15.   S. Devkota, Y, Wang, M. W. Musch, and others, "Dietary-Fat-Induced Taurocholic Acid Promotes Pathobiont Expansion and Colitis in Il10-/- mice." *Nature,* Jul. 5 2012; 487(7405): 104–8, doi:10.1038/nature11225. PubMed PMID: 22722865; PubMed Central PMCID: PMC3393783.

   16.   Honglei Chen, Xuguang Guo, Yikyung Park, and others, "Sweetened-Beverages, Coffee, and Tea in Relation to Depression among Older US Adults (P05.122)," *Neurology,* Feb. 12, 2013; 80(Meeting Abstracts 1): P05.122

   17.   M. Y. Pepino, C. D. Tiemann, B. W. Patterson, and others, "Sucralose Affects Glycemic and Hormonal Responses to an Oral Glucose Load." *Diabetes Care,* Sept. 2013, 36(9): 2530–35, doi:10.2337/dc12-2221. Epub 2013 Apr 30. PubMed PMID: 23633524; PubMed Central PMCID: PMC3747933.

   18.   Hannah Gardener, Tatjana Rundek, Clinton Wright, and others, "Th P55—Soda Consumption and Risk of Vascular Events in the Northern Manhattan Study," P17-Community/Risk Factors Posters II, American Heart Association 2011 International Stroke Conference (http://my.americanheart.org/idc/groups/ahamah-public/@wcm/@sop/@scon/ documents/downloadable/ucm_427795.pdf).

19. "Sugar and Spice and Everything Not So Nice: Spice Allergy Affects Foodies and Cosmetic Users Alike," American College of Allergy, Asthma and Immunology (ACAAI) (Nov. 8, 2012) (no abstract available—http://www.acaai.org/allergist/news/New/Pages/SugarandSpiceandEverythingNotSoNice.aspx).

20. L. DiPietro, A. Gribok, M. S. Stevens, and others, "Three 15-min. Bouts of Moderate Postmeal Walking Significantly Improves 24-h Glycemic Control in Older People at Risk for Impaired Glucose Tolerance, *Diabetes Care*. Oct. 2013; 36(10):3262–68, doi:10.2337/dc13 -0084. Epub 2013 Jun 11. PubMed PMID: 23761134; PubMed Central PMCID: PMC3781561.

21. E. Bonora, "Postprandial Peaks as a Risk Factor for Cardiovascular Disease: Epidemiological Perspectives," *International Journal of Clinical Practice Supplement* 129 (July 2002): 5–11.

22. S. Peele and A. Brodsky, "A General Theory of Addiction," *Love and Addiction*. New York: Taplinger (1975).

23. L. S. Haak and others, "B08 Effectiveness of Team-Based Financial Incentives for Smoking Cessation in the Workplace," Poster Session B, AACR International Conference on Frontiers in Cancer Prevention Research, Oct. 16–19, 2012, Anaheim, California (http://www.aacr.org/home/public--media/aacr-in-the-news.aspx?d=2925).

24. C. Perilloux, J. D. Duntley, and D. M. Buss, "The Costs of Rape," *Archives of Sexual Behavior* 41, no. 5 (Oct. 2012): 1099–106. PubMed PMID: 21975924.

25. S. A. Wilson, L. A. Becker, and R. H. Tinker, "Fifteen-month Follow-up of Eye Movement Desensitization and Reprocessing (EMDR) Treatment for Posttraumatic Stress Disorder and Psychological Trauma," *Journal of Consulting and Clinical Psychology* 65, no. 6 (Dec. 1997): 1047–56. PubMed PMID: 9420367; van der Kolk, J. Spinazzola, M. Blaustein, and others, "A Randomized Clinical Trial of EMDR, Fluoxetine and Pill Placebo in the Treatment of PTSD: Treatment Effects and Long-Term Maintenance," *Journal of Clinical Psychiatry* 68 (2007): 37–46; D. E. Jonas, K. Cusack, C. A. Forneris, and others, "Psychological and Pharmacological Treatments for Adults with Posttraumatic Stress Disorder (PTSD)," Agency for Healthcare Research and Quality (Apr. 2013): http://www.ncbi.nlm.nih.gov/books/NBK137702/ PubMed PMID: 23658937.

26. N. Carmen, "The Power of Rituals in Life, Death, and Business," *Harvard Business School Working Knowledge*, June 2, 2013.

Chapter 6. Week 3: Radiate

1. M. T. Heneka and others, "Locus Ceruleus Controls Alzheimer's Disease Pathology by Modulating Microglial Functions Through Norepinephrine," Proceedings of National Academy of Sciences 107, no. 13 (Mar. 30, 2010): 6058–63, doi:10.1073/pnas.0909586107. Epub 2010 Mar 15. PubMed PMID: 20231476; PubMed Central PMCID: PMC2851853.

2. G. Dawson, "Sleeping Cleans Your Brain," http://real-psychiatry.blogspot .com/2013/10/sleeping-cleans-your-brain.html.

3. B. Dugué and E. Leppänen, "Adaptation Related to Cytokines in Man: Effects of Regular Swimming in Ice-cold Water," *Clinical Physiology* 20, no. 2 (Mar. 2000): 114–21. PubMed PMID: 10735978; P. Huttunen, H. Rintamäki, and J. Hirvonen, "Effect of Regular Winter Swimming on the Activity of the Sympathoadrenal System Before and After a Single Cold Water Immersion," *International Journal of Circumpolar Health* 60, no. 3 (Aug. 2001): 400–406. PubMed PMID: 11590880.

4. L. Rappoport, *How We Eat: Appetite, Culture and the Psychology of Food* (Toronto: ECW Press, 2003).

5. J. Nawijn, M. A. Marchand, R. Veenhoven, and A. J. Vingerhoets, "Vacationers Happier, But Most Not Happier After a Holiday," *Applied Research Quality of Life* 5, no. 1 (Mar. 2010): 35–47.

6. M. E. P. Seligman, T. Rashid, and A. C. Parks, "Positive Psychotherapy." *American Psychologist*, 61 (2006): 774–88.

7. B. J. Fogg, "Fogg Method: 3 Steps to Changing Behavior" http://www.foggmethod .com/

Acknowledgments

Mum, thank you for teaching me that anything is possible. Your unconditional love gave me my confidence and my strength; and to Taki and Nas, thank you for being there, no matter what.

Jerry, thank you for your love and support; and Alexander and Constantine, for sharing your mummy with the world. You are my most important people.

Gwyneth, for your trust and your inspiration as a woman and a mother. I have such respect for your passion and your discipline.

Gideon, my editor, for believing in me and for being such a giving, intuitive leader. Your vision connected all the dots, assembled a great team, and made this book happen.

Mariska, for being my partner in this labor of love and for putting anything I say into excellent words to the point that blows my mind.

Elisabeth and Rupert, for the many years of kindness and support. Your trust and your wisdom are such a gift.

Alicia and Toni, for the constant encouragement and the countless laughs your beautiful friendships have given me.

To my teachers, who brought out the best in me and helped me find my passion at a very young age.

And to the health and healing professionals with whom I've had the pleasure of collaborating, especially Dr. Katja van Herle and Dr. Naji Abumrad, for teaching me so much, for sharing knowledge and resources, and for working together to help our patients make the connection.

And, of course, to all of my beautiful patients and clients, for your loyalty and your vulnerability, for opening yourselves up to new ideas and allowing me into your homes and your lives, for teaching me to be a healer, and for honoring me with your trust. Your talents, strength, and grace inspire and amaze me every day.

Index

Page references followed by *fig* indicate an illustrated figure; followed by *table* indicate a table.

A1C levels, 99
abandonment psychological antidote, 60
acupuncture: considering, 162; Mayo Clinic research on myofacial trigger points corresponding to, 6; self-healing trigger points used during, 122
acute injuries: how both Positive and Negative Feedback start in moment of, 52; Negative Feedback due to, 19; RICE (rest, ice, compression, elevate) for, 192
Adaptive Response: Adam's story on rebuilding his, 32–35; the body's constant tapping into, 56; description of, 11; developing greater resistance to stress through, 54–55; growing stronger because of stress, 18; Holocaust "post-traumatic growth" study on example of, 53; how it uses the SNS, 14–15; how a stable foundation builds resilience of, 40–43; how traditional pain management can interfere with, 11; how yoga manifests the, 154; learning to tap into self-healing, 13; a lifetime of SNS/PNS swings and inability to regulate, 19; making positive choices to wake up your, 36–37; tapping into your innate, 180. *See also* body; pain management; Positive Feedback
addictions: calling in reinforcements to kick your, 159–60; characteristics of those who are able to "quit," 159; Diet Coke, 151; five distinctive characteristics of, 158; Negative Feedback due to unchecked, 20; pattern of inflammatory food, 184–85; release harmful habits and, 158–59. *See also* habits
adrenal glands: cortisol produced by the, 16; HPA axis including the hypothalamus, pituitary gland, and, 15–16
afternoon meditation, 112–13
"aggressively happy" behavior, 5
alcohol, 149, 222*table*
allergies: environmental allergens, 19; as PCOS symptom, 45. *See also* food intolerances/sensitivities
Almond Chocolate Smoothie, 219*table*
almond milk, 191
alpha rhythms, 58
Alzheimer's disease, 73

amygdala: being ruled by our, 60; where we process sensory information into memory and learning, 7
Amy's story: on her successful Positive Feedback program, 22–25; on how her pain affected her, 3–4
anger: Chinese medicine on body's storage of, 6; liver linked to, 9; Positive Feedback remedies for, 244; psychological antidote to, 60; self-healing trigger points on, 126*table*, 129*table*, 244
"angry liver," 203
anxiety: as common reason for seeking medical help, 11; Positive Feedback remedies for, 244–46; psychological antidote to, 60; self-healing trigger point for, 125*table*, 129*table*, 244; spleen linkage to feelings of, 9
Appalachian Trail, 194
artificial creamers, 148
artificial sweeteners, 148
Auschwitz concentration camp, 53
author's story. *See* Vlachonis, Vicky
autonomic nervous system: introduction to the PNS subsystem of, 14, 15*fig*; introduction to the SNS subsystem of, 14, 15*fig*. *See also* nervous system; parasympathetic nervous system (PNS); sympathetic nervous system (SNS)

Baby Boomer health status, 12
baby steps toward goals, 200–201
back-body self-healing trigger points: locations on the body, 123*fig*; working with the, 124*table*–29*table*
back pain: as common reason for seeking medical help, 11; upper, 27*fig*, 31–35, 129*table*. *See also* lower back pain
bagels, 148
baroreflex sensitivity, 22
baths: Epsom salts, 192, 252; lavender, 192, 253; relaxing in a bath, 74; salt-and-pepper, 134–36. *See also* showering
Baumeister, Roy, 20
Berry Smoothie, 218*table*
beta-endorphins, 17–18
beverages: chamomile tea, 73, 222*table*; diseases linked to sugar-sweetened, 59; healing teas, 222*table*; Release (Days 1–7) fall in love with liquids, 145–47; suggested breakfast, 101. *See also* drinking water
Bilophila wadsworthia, 150

Black-Eyed Peas, 239
bladder: infections of the, 184; parasympathetic nervous system (PNS) regulation of, 15*fig*; sympathetic nervous system (SNS) regulation of, 15*fig*
blaming others, 4
bloodflow improvement, 127*table*, 128*table*
blue/purple fruits and vegetables, 189*table*
boar's-hair brush, 131
body: consciously increasing the flow of natural painkillers of the, 6; constantly tapping into Adaptive Response, 56; Dr. Still's belief in self-healing power of the, 51–52; effects of chronic inflammation on the, 10–11; illustration of self-healing trigger points on the, 123; imprint of negative thought carried throughout your, 8–9; law of inertia on resting, 52; learning to listen to your, 41–43; possible reactions to the Release Meal Plan by your, 152–53; Reflect phase to reconnect with your physical, 57–58. *See also* Adaptive Response; Maladaptive Response
body brushes, 131
Body Family Tree: how to create your, 86–87; how to effectively use your, 87, 90–91; sample of your, 88*fig*–89*fig*
Body Map, 85–86
Body Map Template, 85, 86*fig*
body scan for pain, 155
Body Timeline: description and benefits of, 91–92; example of a, 92*fig*–93*fig*; Lisa's, 203–4; multifold purpose of, 92; process of creating your, 93–95
brain: amygdala of the, 7, 60; Brown University study on meditation benefits to the, 40; cortex of the, 7; HPA axis of the, 15–17; hypothalamus of the, 7, 15–16, 129*table*; impact of chronic stress on the, 16; plaque build-up in the, 53; prefrontal cortex (PFC) of the, 61, 180; SNS/PNS swings experienced by the, 16–19; "volume knob" for controlling alpha rhythms of your, 58
brain-derived neurotrophic factor (BDNF), 62
brainstorming Radiant life, 198–201
Brazil nuts, 148
bread: Positive Feedback complex carbohydrates, 188*table*; suggested breakfast, 101
breakfast meal plans: Radiate Meal Plan, 216*table*–17*table*, 220*table*; Release (Days 1–3) Liver Flush, 142–43, 212*table*; suggested smoothies for, 101; suggestions for a Reflection, 100–101
breathing exercises: during meditation, 110–11; nine-point meditation and deep, 134; relax and release tension with deep, 21–22; Tibetan Rites finished with deep, 83
British School of Osteopathy, 43
Brown, Brené, 36
brown fat cells, 183

Brown University, 40
buried emotions, 6
Butterflied Roast Chicken, 230

Cabrito with Prunes, 231
California Fresh Salad, 224
candy, 149
cashew nuts, 148
Cats cast members, 47–48
Centers for Disease Control and Prevention (CDC), 11–12
chamomile tea, 73, 222*table*
champagne, 222*table*
Check-ins: are you ready to live in Positive Feedback for life?, 202–7; are you ready to Radiate?, 173; are you ready to Release?, 114
chickenpox virus, 4
Chickpea Salad, 241–42
childhood: EMDR therapy to release trauma from, 164–66; how a stable foundation builds life-long health, 39–43; how we "install" our emotional triggers during, 8; identifying your passion by examining memories from your, 195–96; learning the power of food to hurt or heal during, 41–43; Negative Feedback due to unresolved trauma from, 20; Radiant Deep Dive by recalling happiest day during, 197–98, 205; rituals used to release past trauma from, 167–71
chili powder, 149
Chinese medicine: on the gallbladder point, 124*table*; on the heart point, 127*table*; on where anger is stored in the body, 6; on yin and yang, 129*table*
chiropractors, 162
chocolate, 222*table*
Chödrön, Pema, 51
choices: to make positive, 36–37; psychic effects of taking control through good, 61; Reflect*Release*Radiate sequence for making, 52; understanding the power of, 53–55
chronic neurological problems, 11
chronic stress: impact on the HPA axis, 16–17; Negative Feedback due to unmanaged, 20; post-traumatic stress disorder, 165–66
coffee, 148
colds and coughs remedies, 246
cold sores, 42, 46
compassion, 65, 202
complex carbohydrates: food sources of, 188*table*; Positive Feedback To-Go Plan for lowering intake of, 192
constipation: changing food intake to improve, 184–86; PCOS symptom of, 44, 46; self-healing trigger points to help with, 126*table*, 128*table*

contentment system: how the Positive
Feedback plan can strengthen your, 201–2;
how Radiant relationships strengthen your,
201–2; when the PNS slows us down, 18
cortex, 7
cortisol hormone, 16
cow's milk, 148
cranial sacral therapy, 73
C-reactive protein, 73
curcumin, 143–44
Current Directions in Psychological Science, 135
cytokines, 183

daily naps, 136–38, 192
daily reflection exercise, 83, 182
dairy products, 149–51
Daring Greatly (Brown), 36
decision making: for positive choices, 36–37,
52–55, 61; Reflect*Release*Radiate sequence used for, 55
deep breathing exercises: during nine-point
meditation, 134; to relax and release tension, 21–22; Tibetan Rites finished with, 83
Deep Dive, 196–98, 205
depression: as common reason for seeking medical help, 11; Positive Feedback
remedies for, 244–46; self-healing trigger
points for anxiety and, 125*table*, 129*table*,
244. *See also* sadness
desserts: Radiate Meal Plan special treats,
222*table*; Release (Days 1–3) Liver
Flush, 143
detoxification: Release Meal Plan for, 138–52,
185; Release of toxic inflammatory foods,
147–52, 212*table*–13*table*
Diabetes Care journal, 153
diabetes Type 2, 59, 214
diaphragm release point, 125*table*
diet: keeping Food Diary on your, 95–97;
making changes during Radiate phase,
184–89; Mediterranean, 185–86; Positive Feedback complex carbohydrates to
include in, 188*table*; Positive Feedback
proteins to include in, 187*table*–88*table*;
Positive Feedback vegetables and fruits to
include in, 189*table*; reintroducing reactive
foods to your, 190, 193; Release Meal Plan,
59, 138–53, 185; travel/jet lag remedies
and suggested, 256–57. *See also* foods;
poor diet
Diet Coke, 151, 205
diet soda, 59, 74, 151–52, 205
differential diagnosis, 243
digestive upset: inflammatory foods associated with, 140; leaky gut syndrome, 19;
self-healing trigger points for improving,
124*table*–29*table*

dinner meal plans: Radiate Meal Plan,
217*table*, 221*table*; Release (Day 1–7)
release the toxic inflammatory foods, 143,
213*table*; Release (Days 1–3) Liver Flush,
143; Release (Days 1–7) fall in love with
liquids, 143, 213*table*
diseases: differential diagnosis of, 243; Dr.
Still's approach to, 51–52; emotional pain
making us more vulnerable to, 7; heart disease, 59, 102, 214; osteopathy's self-healing
approach to, 43; Type 2 diabetes, 59, 214.
See also illness
drinking water: with juice of half a lemon,
76–77, 146; reverse osmosis filter installed
to protect your, 146–47; stopping three
hours before bed, 73; 316 chemicals found
in U.S., 146. *See also* beverages
drug overdose deaths, 11–12
dry brushing: description and function
of, 130–31; how to apply to your body,
131–33; for lymphatic drainage, 132*fig*;
during Radiate phase, 182

eczema: inflammatory foods associated with,
140; as PCOS symptom, 45, 46. *See also*
skin issues
edema: inflammatory foods associated with,
140; self-healing trigger points in case
of, 28*table*
eggplant, 148
eggs: protein source from, 187*table*; suggested
breakfast, 101
Egg-White Frittata with Feta Cheese and
Chives, 230–31
EMDR therapy, 162, 164–66, 204
emotional eating, 19
emotional pain: connection between physical
and, 7–10; making us more vulnerable to
diseases, 7; psychological antidotes to common types of, 60*table*. *See also* pain
emotional triggers: how we "install" our, 8;
list of typical SNS triggers, 17
emotions: all the parts of the brain that intersect when experiencing, 7; anger, 6, 9, 60,
126*table*, 129*table*, 244; anxiety, 9, 11, 60,
125*table*, 129*table*, 244–46; fear, 9–10, 19,
65–66; normal nature of, 5; organ-emotion
linkages, 9; problems as caused by buried,
6; sadness, 9, 20, 60, 125*table*
emotion self-care techniques, 54
emotion work: Radiate phase, 195–202,
205; Reflect phase positive emotions, 102;
Release phase positive emotions,
155–63
endocrine system: Adaptive Response impact
on the, 54; hypothalamus messages sent
to the, 16
energy drinks, 148

energy point, 126*table*
the engaged life, 199
environmental allergens, 19
Environmental Working Group, 146–47
Epsom salts bath, 192, 252
European School of Osteopathy, 43
evening meditation, 113–14
eye motion desensitization and reprocessing
    (EMDR) therapy, 162, 164–66, 204
The Eye of Revelation (Kelder), 77
eyes: parasympathetic nervous system (PNS)
    regulation of, 15*fig*; sympathetic nervous
    system (SNS) regulation of, 15*fig*

family history: Body Family Tree based on
    your, 86–91; physical and emotional legacy
    carried from our, 7–8, 201–2
fast foods, 148
fear: connection between feeling pain and,
    9–10; kidney linked to feeling, 9; Negative
    Feedback due to continuous, 19; Radiate
    phase to let go of your, 65–66
fertility issues, 129*table*
fight-or-flight reaction: childhood patterns
    of, 8; PNS as the break slowing down the,
    18; the SNS "drive" response to, 14–15,
    16–17, 18
fish (oily), 187*table*, 204
fish recipes: Mediterranean Salsa (for fish),
    234; Oven-Baked Branzino with Cherry
    Tomato and Caper Salsa, 228–29; Pan-
    Grilled Ahi Tuna or Mahi-Mahi, 229
flaxseed, 147
flu remedies, 246–47
Food Diary: description and contents of, 95;
    reactive foods identified in your, 190, 193;
    sample of before and after, 96*fig*; when to
    record in your, 97
food intolerances/sensitivities: connection be-
    tween PCOS and, 45–46; identifying your,
    141; Negative Feedback due to continuous,
    19; spices as cause of, 152. *See also* aller-
    gies; inflammatory foods
foods: from Grandma's kitchen, 41–43, 47;
    lesson on power to hurt or heal of, 41–43;
    Positive Feedback complex carbohydrates,
    188*table*; Positive Feedback proteins,
    187*table*–88*table*; Positive Feedback veg-
    etables and fruits, 189*table*; reintroducing
    reactive, 190, 193. *See also* diet; inflamma-
    tory foods; Release Meal Plan
forgiveness: overcoming your fears, ac-
    knowledging pain, and, 166–67; releasing
    your past via ritual in order to engage in,
    167–71; religious rituals for, 168; visualiza-
    tion in order to release, 171–73
Frankl, Viktor, 53
French Green Beans, 238

Fresh Spinach Salad, 225
front-body self-healing trigger points: loca-
    tion on the body, 123*fig*; working with,
    124*table*–29*table*
Frontiers of Human Neuroscience, 58
Fruit Salad, 226
function self-care techniques, 54

gallbladder point, 124*table*
Garlic and Chili Broccolini (Long-Stem
    Broccoli), 237–38
Gilbert, Paul, 14
glial cells, 73
glucose build-up, 53
gluten-based food products, 148
glymphatic system, 73
goals: for each stage of
    Reflect*Release*Radiate sequence, 52;
    identifying your passion to establish new,
    195–99; Release phase as most popular and
    primary, 58–60; setting Radiate positive
    motion, 194–95; taking baby steps toward
    your, 200–201
goat milk, 187*table*, 192
gout, 59
grains, 188*table*
Grandma's kitchen food, 41–43, 47
Greek Burgers, 233
Greek Goddess Salad, 225
green vegetables: Positive Feedback, 189*table*;
    Release Meal Plan, 213*table*. *See also*
    specific recipe
grief-lungs linkage, 9
Guacamole recipe, 242
"gut feelings," 9

habits: calling in reinforcements to kick
    your harmful, 159–60; consciously
    choosing to practice good, 54–55;
    Reflect*Release*Radiate sequence used for
    deciding on, 55; release harmful, 158–59.
    See also addictions
hangover remedies, 247–48
Hanson, Rick, 14, 60
happiness: Lisa's story on creating a medita-
    tion to visualize, 205; meditation on confi-
    dence, self-belief, and, 207; the three ways
    to develop path for, 199
"happy" oils, 84
Hardwiring Happiness (Hanson), 14
harmful habits. *See* addictions
Harvard study, 65
headaches: as common reason for seeking
    medical help, 11; Positive Feedback rem-
    edies for, 248–49; self-healing trigger point
    for, 129*table*, 248
healing teas, 222*table*

health: author's story on turnaround from pain to, 43–47; how a stable foundation maintains good, 40–43; muscular, 20, 127*table*, 140; skeletal, 20

health modalities: exploring a new, 160–63; suggestions for some to consider, 162

heart: parasympathetic nervous system (PNS) regulation of, 15*fig*; sympathetic nervous system (SNS) regulation of, 15*fig*

heart disease: Mayo Clinic research on exercise and, 102; modern increase in, 214; sugar-sweetened beverages linked to, 59

heart point, 127*table*

high-fructose corn syrup, 139

hippocampus: HPA axis role of the, 15–17; meditation impact on the, 60

hip self-healing trigger points, 126*table*

holistic nutritionist, 162

Holocaust "post-traumatic growth" study, 53

HPA axis: chronic stress impact on the, 16–17; description of the, 15–16

Humulus lupulus (hops fruit), 75

hydration. *See* drinking water

hyperactivity, 140

hypnotherapist, 162

hypothalamus: connecting with endocrine system and the gut organs, 7; HPA axis made up of pituitary gland, adrenal glands and, 15–16; regulation functions of the, 16; self-healing trigger points for the, 129*table*

illness: differential diagnosis of, 243; osteopathy's self-healing approach to, 43; spinal column as "decoder ring" to diagnose, 13. *See also* diseases; Positive Feedback remedies

immune system: how shingles can result from overtaxed, 4; hypothalamus messages sent to the, 16; legacy carried from our parents that affect the, 7–8

Immunology journal, 149

inflammation: effects of chronic, 10–11; evidenced on the surface of the body, 10; making positive choices for tamping down your, 37; as primary physical mechanism of Negative Feedback, 179; tumor necrosis factor and C-reactive protein markers for, 73

inflammatory foods: common symptoms associated with, 140; common types of, 148–49; dairy and red meat, 149–51; diet soda as, 59, 74, 151–52; high-fructose corn syrup, 139; pattern of addictions to, 184–85; wheat products, 149. *See also* food intolerances/sensitivities; foods; poor diet

injuries: how both Positive and Negative Feedback start in moment of, 52; Negative Feedback due to, 19; RICE (rest, ice, compression, elevate) for, 192

insomnia: consequences of chronic sleep deprivation and, 72; self-healing trigger points to help with, 126*table*, 128; tips to avoid, 73–75

insulin resistance, 19

intestines: parasympathetic nervous system (PNS) regulation of, 15*fig*; sympathetic nervous system (SNS) regulation of, 15*fig*

Jawbone UP, 74

Jeffers, Susan, 65

Jennifer's story, 63–65*table*

Jenny's Greek Bolognese Sauce, 232–33

Jerry's Crab Salad, 226

Jewish Polish population study, 53

joint disorders: as common reason for seeking medical help, 11; inflammatory foods associated with, 140

Journal of the Academy of Nutrition and Dietetics, 99

Journal of Affective Disorders, 98

Journal of Neuroscience, 58

Kabat-Zinn, Jon, 39

Kale Smoothie, 219*table*

Kelder, Peter, 77

Kerry's story, 116–18

ketchup, 148

kidneys: fear linked to, 9; sympathetic nervous system (SNS) regulation of, 15*fig*

Kierkegaard, Søren, 71

Kiwi Lemon Smoothie, 219*table*

knee self-healing trigger points, 127*table*, 128*table*

lavender bath, 192, 253

leaky gut syndrome, 19

lean meat, 187*table*

lean poultry, 187*table*

Learned Optimism and Authentic Happiness (Seligman), 198

leg self-healing trigger points, 127*table*, 128*table*

lemon water, 76–77, 146

lethargy-inflammatory foods association, 140

letting it go: faith working in tandem with treatments for, 119–20; pretreatment ritual before treatments for, 119; treatments to help you in, 118–19

life expectancy decline, 12

limbic system, 7

The Lion King cast members, 47–48

Lisa's story, 203–5

listening to pain, 3–4, 163

liver: anger linked to, 9; "angry liver" condition of the, 203; parasympathetic nervous system (PNS) regulation of, 15*fig*; sympathetic nervous system (SNS) regulation of, 15*fig*; toxins build up in the, 53

Liver Flush, 142–45, 212–13

Liver Flush Smoothie, 144–45, 212*table*

live yogurt, 187*table*

lower back pain: common profile of, 28–31; inflammatory foods associated with, 140; Jennifer's Positive Feedback profile on her, 63–65*table*; physical and emotional causes in men, 27*fig*; physical and emotional causes in women, 27*fig*; Positive Feedback remedies for, 249–50; Sarah's story on her, 29–31; self-healing trigger points for, 126*table*, 127*table*, 128*table*, 249; as signal to change, 162–63. *See also* back pain

low libido: Positive Feedback remedies for, 250–51; self-healing trigger points for, 127*table*, 129*table*, 250

lunch meal plans: Radiate Meal Plan, 217*table*, 221*table*; Release (Day 1–7) release the toxic inflammatory foods, 213*table*; Release (Days 1–3) Liver Flush, 143, 213*table*; Release (Days 1–7) fall in love with liquids, 143, 213*table*

lungs: parasympathetic nervous system (PNS) regulation of, 15*fig*; sadness, worry, grief linked to, 9; sympathetic nervous system (SNS) regulation of, 15*fig*

lymphatic drainage: dry brushing for, 132*fig*; self-healing trigger points to help with, 125*table*, 126*table*, 127*table*

lymphatic system: description and function of the, 130–31; draining the toxins from your, 125*table*, 126*table*, 127*table*, 1323*fig*

lymph nodes, 53

main dish recipes: Butterflied Roast Chicken, 230; Cabrito with Prunes, 231; Egg-White Frittata with Feta Cheese and Chives, 230–31; Greek Burgers, 233; Jenny's Greek Bolognese Sauce, 232–33; Mediterranean Salsa (for fish), 234; Oven-Baked Branzino with Cherry Tomato and Caper Salsa, 228–29; Pan-Grilled Ahi Tuna or Mahi-Mahi, 229; Roast Chicken/Turkey with Figs, 232

Maladaptive Response, 18–19. *See also* body

Man's Search for Meaning (Frankl), 53

manual therapy, 43

margarine, 148

massage: considering treatment of, 162; "happy" oils used for, 84; as Morning Glory routine, 84, 130; self-healing trigger points used during, 122; tummy, 182, 183–84

Mayo Clinic research: on acupuncture points corresponding to myofacial trigger points, 6; on exercise and heart disease, 102

mayonnaise, 148

meal plans. *See* Positive Feedback meal plans

the meaningful life, 199

meat: lean, 187*table*; processed, 148; red, 149–51

meditation: afternoon, 112–13; breathing exercise during, 110–11; Brown University study on benefits of, 40; on confidence, happiness, and self-belief, 207; creating your own release through visualization and, 163, 166–67; evening, 113–14; health benefits of, 39–40, 60; increasing compassion through, 65; Lisa's story on creating a happiness, 205; mindful eating and grateful, 98; morning, 84, 111–12; Morning Glory ritual ended with a morning, 84; nine-point, 130, 133–34; purpose and benefits of, 108–11; study on alpha rhythms and, 58; Wake Forest University study on pain management using, 109. *See also* physical exercise

Mediterranean Salsa (for fish), 234

Mediterranean style of eating, 185–86

Mednick, Sara, 137

Melissa's story, 175–79

memory: amygdala where sensory information is processed into, 7; how new experiences may retrigger an old, 92; identifying your passion by examining your childhood, 195–96; Radiant Deep Dive by recalling happiest day as a child, 197–98, 205; trauma and misfiled, 164–66

menstrual pain remedies, 251–52

meta-cognition, 62

mid-back pain: emotional causes of, 27*fig*; physical causes of, 27*fig*

milk: almond, 191; cow, 148; goat, 187*table*, 192

mindful eating: description of, 97; eating as slowly as possible for, 99; grateful meditation before, 98; ground rules for, 98; suggestions for a Reflection breakfast, 100–101

mindfulness: as the mind task of Week 1: Reflect, 71; training us to be present in the moment, 57; as way of being, 39

moderation, 214

Monica's story, 55

Morning Glory ritual: consider adding to evening routine, 74; daily restoration through the, 206; description of, 75; dry brushing, 130–34; ending it with a morning meditation, 84, 111–12; nine-point meditation, 130, 133–34; Radiate at-a-glance, 182; Reflect-Week at-a-glance, 76; Release-Week at-a-glance, 130; salt-and-pepper bath, 134–36; shower, dry, and massage your body, 83–84, 130; Tibetan Rites as part of the, 76, 78–82, 130, 182; tips for using the, 75–77. *See also* rituals

morning meditation, 84, 111–12

motion self-care techniques, 54

muscular health: inflammatory foods associated with poor, 140; Negative Feedback
impact on, 20; self-healing trigger points to
help with, 127*table*
mushrooms, 148
myofacial trigger points: learning to release
pain using your, 6; Mayo Clinic research
on acupuncture points corresponding to, 6.
See also self-healing trigger points

nap (daily), 136–38, 192
National Health Service (UK), 44
Nature journal, 150
naturopathic doctor, 162
neck pain: emotional causes of, 27*fig*; physical
cause of, 27*fig*; Positive Feedback remedies
for, 252–53; self-healing trigger points
for, 252
Negative Feedback: chronic stress and
cycle of, 15–17; conditions that trigger or
perpetuate, 19–21; emotional responses
during experience of, 4–5; how pain medication often leads to, 11; inflammation as
the primary physical mechanism of, 179;
keeping you trapped in pain, 53; negative
self-talk that is part of, 61; premature aging legacy of lifetime of, 19; three steps to
interrupt the loop of, 49; understood as a
voluntary state, 35
Negative Feedback liberation: radiate into
your best life, 49; reflect on the pain step,
49; release the guilt, 49
negative self-talk, 61
negative thoughts: carried throughout our
body, 8–9; visualize and wash away, 133
"negativity bias," 20–21
Nepali pranayama study, 21
nervous system: central, 14; imprint of negative
thought carried by your, 8–9; peripheral, 14;
understanding how it reacts to pain, 13. *See
also* autonomic nervous system
The New York Times, reporting on drug overdoses from pain medication, 12
Nin, Anaïs, 115
nine-point meditation, 130, 133–34
NutriBullet, 147
nuts: to avoid, 148; Positive Feedback proteins, 187*table*; Positive Feedback To-Go
Plan on snacking with, 192; Release Meal
Plan, 213*table*
Nutty Smoothie, 218*table*

oatmeal, 101
obesity/toxic visceral fat, 19
oily fish, 187*table*, 205
omega-3 fatty acids: food sources of, 185,
187*table*, 214; Negative Feedback due to
deficiency in, 19

Omega Smoothie, 218*table*
oranges, 148
orange/yellow fruits and vegetables, 189*table*
organ-emotion linkages, 9
organic almond milk, 191
osteopathy: description of self-healing
approach of, 43; differential diagnosis
approach by, 243; not available throughout
the U.S., 161; Positive Feedback program
powered by the core mechanisms of,
51–52
Oven-Baked Branzino with Cherry Tomato
and Caper Salsa, 228–29
OxyContin overdoses, 11–12
oxytocin hormone, 138

Pacific Crest Trail, 194
pain: ability of meditation to relieve, 109–10;
author's story on turnaround to health
from, 43–47; Body Timeline to recall
your, 94–95; connection between emotional and physical, 7–10; forgiveness for
your, 166–67, 171–73; how the nervous
system reacts to pain, 13; learning to
listen to what it is saying to you, 3–4,
163; letting go of the, 118–20; Negative
Feedback keeping you trapped in, 53;
quick body scan for habitual offenders
causing, 155; referred, 26; silent prayer
during shower to wash away the, 133;
understanding the reason for your, 5. *See
also* emotional pain; trauma
pain location: description of, 26; location of
pain and its possible causes, 27*fig*; lower
back pain, 27*fig*, 28–31; neck pain, 27*fig*;
upper back pain, 27*fig*, 31–35
pain management: meditation used as,
109–10; myofacial trigger points for pain
release and, 125*table*; traditional allopathic
approach to, 11. *See also* Adaptive Response
pain medications: CDC on increasing death
rate from, 11–12; often leading to Negative
Feedback, 11; pain management using,
109–10; used by Royal Ballet School
dancers, 47–48
Pan-Grilled Ahi Tuna or Mahi-Mahi, 229
panic attack self-healing trigger point,
125*table*
pan metron ariston (everything in moderation), 214
parasympathetic nervous system (PNS): beta-
endorphins released by, 17–18; description
of, 14; functioning as the relaxation response, 18; heavily influenced by thoughts,
20; preparing for pregnancy by resettling,
205; regulation of functioning organs by,
15*fig*; working to strengthen the, 21–22,
180. *See also* autonomic nervous system

parents: Body Family Tree based on family history of, 86–91; physical and emotional legacy carried from our, 7–8, 201–2

passion: baby steps to fulfilling your, 200–201; as core of radiant living, 202; developing path to happiness and your, 199; identifying by examining childhood memories, 195–96

pasta, 188*table*

peanuts, 148

Peas and Artichoke Hearts, 239–40

perimenopausal issues, self-healing trigger points for low, 172327*table*

pessimism psychological antidote, 60

physical exercise: Mayo Clinic research on heart disease and, 102; Negative Feedback due to continuous lack of, 19; Radiate phase and challenging new goals for, 194–95; Tibetan Rites, 52, 74, 76–83, 102, 130, 194; walking, 153–54, 192; yoga, 154. *See also* meditation; Positive Feedback exercises

pickles, 148

pineapples, 147

pistachios, 148

pituitary gland, 15–16

plaque build-up, 53

the pleasant life, 199

polycystic ovary syndrome (PCOS): connection between food sensitivities and, 45–46; diagnosis of, 44; turnaround from pain to health, 45–47

poor diet: how it contributes to eczema, allergies, and skin issues, 45; insomnia relationship to, 74–75; Negative Feedback due to continuous, 19. *See also* diet; inflammatory foods

positive emotion (Radiate phase): brainstorming your Radiate life, 198–99; Deep Dive, 196–98, 205; identifying your passion, 195–96; investing in Radiant relationships, 201–2; taking baby steps toward your new goals during, 200–201

positive emotion self care: description of, 54; Positive Feedback category of, 54; Radiate phase, 195–202, 205; Reflect phase, 102; Release phase, 155–73

positive emotion (Reflect phase), 102

positive emotion (Release phase): call in reinforcements, 159–60; explore a new health modality, 160–63; issues to consider for, 155–56; meditation/visualization, 163, 166–67; release harmful habits, 158–59; release time-wasters on your Time Audit, 156–58; release your past via ritual, 167–71; visualize forgiveness and release, 171–73

Positive Feedback: emotional responses of, 22; how it can make you well, 35–37; making positive choices to move toward, 36–37;

Reflect*Release*Radiate sequence of the, 52. *See also* Adaptive Response

Positive Feedback cycle, 36

Positive Feedback exercises: breathing, 21–22, 83, 110–11, 134; daily reflection, 83, 182; Release the Time-Wasters exercise, 117, 156–58; suggestions for getting the most out of, 67. *See also* physical exercise

Positive Feedback meal plans: health benefits of the, 211; my mum's voice: moderation, 214; my mum's voice: raise your glass, 211; Positive Feedback To-Go Plan, 192; Radiate Meal Plan, 185–89*table*, 190, 193, 214–22*table*; Release Meal Plan, 59, 128–53, 185, 212*table*-14

Positive Feedback prescription, 64*table*-65*table*

Positive Feedback profiles, 63–65*table*

Positive Feedback program: Amy's story on her success with, 22–25; four self-care technique categories of the, 54; Monica's story on her experience with, 55; osteopathic treatments as powering the, 51–52; power of choice and the, 53–55; preparing to start the, 66–67; Week 1: Reflect, 71–114; Week 2: Release, 115–73; Week 3: Radiate, 175–207. *See also* Reflect*Release*Radiate sequence

Positive Feedback program Week 1: Reflect phase: affirmations and meditation, 108–14; Body Family Tree, 86–91; Body Map, 85–86*fig*; Body Timeline, 91–95; check-in: are you ready to move to Release?, 114; daily reflection exercise, 83; Food Diary, 95–97; mindful eating, 97–101; Morning Flory ritual, 75–85; positive emotions during the, 102; positive motion used during the, 102; positive self-talk used during the, 103–5, 107; positive structures used during the, 85–95; sufficient quality sleep, 72–75; Time Audit, 106*fig*-8

Positive Feedback program Week 2: Release phase: check-in: are you ready to move to Radiate?, 173; importance of this phase, 115–16; Kerry's story on, 116–18; letting it go, 118–20; Morning Glory ritual at-a-glance during the, 130; positive emotion during the, 155–73; positive functions during the, 138–53; positive structure during the, 120–38; quick body scan for habitual offenders during the, 155; Release Meal Plan for detoxification, 138–52, 185, 212*table*-14; self-healing trigger points used during the, 121–29*table*

Positive Feedback program Week 3: Radiate phase: check-in: are you ready to live in Positive Feedback for life?, 202–7; finding your purpose during the, 181; Melissa's story on journey to the, 175–79; positive emotion during the, 195–202; positive

Positive Feedback program Week 3 *(cont.)*
motion during the, 193–95; positive
structure during the, 181–93; a quick scan
of where we are when starting the, 179–80;
Radiate Meal Plan, 185–89*table*, 190, 193,
214–22*table*; what to expect during the,
180–81
Positive Feedback recipes: main dishes,
228–34; salads, 224–26; side dishes,
234–42; soups, 227–28
Positive Feedback remedies: for anger, 244;
for anxiety and depression, 244–46; for
colds and coughs, 246; differential diagnosis approach of, 243; for flu, 246–47; for
hangover, 247–48; for headache, 248–49;
for low back pain, 249–50; for low libido,
250–51; for menstrual pain, 251–52; for
neck pain, 252–53; for sore throat, 253–54;
for thyroid, 254; for travel and jet lag,
255–57. *See also* illness; self-healing trigger points
Positive Feedback self-care categories: positive emotion, 54, 102, 155–73, 195–202,
205; positive function, 54, 95–101, 138–52,
184–89*table*; positive motion, 52, 54, 74,
76–83, 102, 153–54, 193–95; positive structure, 54, 85–95, 120–28, 182–84
Positive Feedback supplements, 215
Positive Feedback To-Go Meal Plan, 192
positive function self-care: Radiate phase,
184–89*table*; Reflect phase, 95–101; Release phase, 138–52, 185. *See also* Positive
Feedback self-care categories
Positive function (Radiate phase): making
changes in diet intake, 184–86; Positive
Feedback complex carbohydrates, 188*table*;
Positive Feedback proteins, 187*table*–
88*table*; Positive Feedback vegetables and
fruits, 189*table*
Positive function (Reflect phase): Food Diary,
95–97; mindful eating, 97–101; purpose of
establishing, 95
Positive function (Release phase): Release Meal
Plan for detoxification, 138–42, 185; Release
Meal Plans (Days 1–3), 142–45; Release
Meal Plans (Days 1–7), 145–47; Release toxic inflammatory foods (Days 1–7), 147–49;
troublesome categories of food, 149–52
Positive motion (Radiate phase): activities and
goals to consider for, 194–95; improved
physical condition during the, 193–94
positive motion (Reflect phase): overview of
the, 102; Release phase, 153–54; Tibetan
Rites, 52, 74, 76–83, 102
positive motion (Release phase): take a quick
stroll, 153–54; yoga, 154
positive motion self-care: description of the,
54; Radiate phase, 193–95; Reflect phase,
52, 74, 76–83, 102; Release phase, 153–54

positive psychology, 198–99
positive self-talk, 103–7
positive structure self-care: description of,
54; Radiate phase, 182–84; Reflect phase,
85–95; Release phase, 120–38
positive structure (Radiate phase): alternating hot and cold rinses, 182–83; Morning
Glory ritual at-a-glance, 182; tummy massage, 182, 183–84
positive structure (Reflect phase): Body Family Tree, 86–91; Body Map, 85–86*fig*; Body
Timeline, 91–95
positive structure (Release phase): issues to
consider for establishing, 120–21; Morning
Glory enhancements, 130–38; self-healing
trigger points, 121–29*table*
post-traumatic stress disorder, 165–66. *See
also* stress
potatoes: Release Meal Plan, 213*table*;
sweet, 213*table*; Sweet Potato Mash, 241;
white, 149
poultry protein, 187*table*
poultry recipes: Butterflied Roast Chicken,
230; Greek Burgers, 233; Roast Chicken/
Turkey with Figs, 232
power of choice, 53–54
pranayama meditative exercise, 21
prayer (silent), 133
prefrontal cortex (PFC), 61, 180
pregnancy, 205
premenstrual self-healing trigger points,
126*table*, 128*table*
processed meats, 148
proteins: complete-protein combinations,
188*table*; Positive Feedback, 187*table*–
88*table*; Positive Feedback To-Go Plan on
increasing, 192
Protein Shake, 218*table*
psychological antidotes, 60
Pumpkin (or Sweet potato) Soup, 227
purple/blue vegetables, 189*table*

Radiant Deep Dive, 196–98, 205
Radiant living: check-in: are you ready to
live in Positive Feedback for life?, 202–7;
passion as the core and goal of, 195–96,
199–202; Radiant relationships as part of
your, 201–2
Radiant relationships, 201–2
Radiate Meal Plan: breakfasts, 216*table*–
17*table*, 220*table*; comparing the Release
Meal Plan and, 185; description of the,
185–86, 214–15; healing teas, 222*table*;
lunches and dinners, 217*table*, 221*table*;
more meal choices under the, 215; Positive
Feedback complex carbohydrates used in,
188*table*; Positive Feedback proteins used
in, 187*table*–88*table*; Positive Feedback

vegetables and fruits, 189*table*; reintroducing reactive foods, 190, 193; snacks,
216*table*–17*table*, 221*table*; special treats,
222*table*; supplements, 215
Radiate phase: baby steps toward your goals,
200–201; brainstorming your Radiant
life, 198–201; check-in: are you ready
to live in Positive Feedback for life?,
202–7; check-in: are you ready to move
to Radiate?, 173; Deep Dive, 196–98, 205;
finding your purpose during the, 181;
investing in Radiant relationships during,
201–2; Jennifer's individualized Positive
Feedback prescription for, 65*table*; Morning Glory ritual at-a-glance, 182; overview of the, 61–62, 65–66; Radiate Meal
Plan, 185–89*table*, 190, 193, 214–22*table*;
what you can expect during the,
180–81. *See also* Reflect*Release*Radiate
sequence
rape victims, 165
Reactive foods, 190, 193
recipes. *See* Positive Feedback recipes
red fruits and vegetables, 189*table*
red meat, 149–51
referred pain, 26
Reflect*Release*Radiate sequence: used as
decision-making technique, 55; Negative
Feedback liberation step of, 49; overview of
the three steps of, 56–66; pleasure of seeing someone successfully go through the,
202–7; ultimate goal of each stage of the,
52. *See also* Positive Feedback program;
specific step
Reflect phase: affirmations and meditation, 108–14; Body Family Tree, 86–91;
Body Map, 85–86*fig*; Body Timeline,
91–95; check-in: are you ready to move to
Release?, 114; daily reflection exercise, 83;
Food Diary, 95–97; get sufficient quality
sleep during the, 72–75; Jennifer's individualized Positive Feedback prescription
for, 64*table*; mindful eating, 97–101; Morning Flory ritual, 75–85; overview of the,
56–58; positive self-talk during the, 103–5,
107; to reconnect with your physical self,
57–58; Time Audit, 106*fig*–8. *See also*
Reflect*Release*Radiate sequence
reflexologist, 162
rejection psychological antidote, 60
Release Meal Plan: comparing the Radiate
Meal Plan and, 185; description and benefits of the, 59; description and detoxification using the, 138–42, 185; possible body
reactions to the, 152–53; Release (Day
1–7) release the toxic inflammatory foods,
147–52, 212*table*–13*table*; Release (Days
1–3) cleanse via a Liver Flush, 142–45,
212*table*–13*table*; Release (Days 1–7) fall

in love with liquids, 145–47, 212*table*–
13*table*. *See also* foods
Release phase: check-in: are you ready to
Radiate?, 114; daily nap, 136–38; drink
lemon water, 76–77, 146; dry brushing,
130–33; importance of the, 115–16; Jennifer's individualized Positive Feedback
prescription for, 64*table*; Kerry's story on,
116–18; letting it go during the, 118–20;
Morning Glory ritual at-a-glance, 130;
nine-point meditation, 133–34; overview of the, 58–60, 61; as primary goal
of most patients, 58–60; quick body scan
for habitual offenders during the, 155;
Release Meal Plan for detoxification,
138–52, 185, 212*table*–14; salt-and-
pepper bath, 134–36; self-healing trigger
points used during, 121–29*table*. *See also*
Reflect*Release*Radiate sequence
Release the Time-Wasters exercise: description and benefits of, 156–58; Kerry's story
on her, 117
remedies. *See* Positive Feedback remedies
resveratrol, 143
reverse osmosis filter, 146–47
rice, 188*table*
RICE (rest, ice, compression, elevate), 192
rituals: closure through a "proper burial,"
171; letting it go and pretreatment, 119;
release your past via, 167–71; religion and
forgiveness, 168. *See also* Morning Glory
ritual
Roast Chicken/Turkey with Figs, 232
Royal Ballet School, 47
Rozin, Paul, 21

sadness: linkage between lungs and, 9;
Negative Feedback due to unrelenting, 20;
psychological antidote to, 60; self-healing
trigger point for, 125*table*. *See also* depression
salad recipes: California Fresh Salad, 224;
Fresh Spinach Salad, 225; Fruit Salad, 226;
Greek Goddess Salad, 225; Jerry's Crab
Salad, 226
salivary glands: parasympathetic nervous system (PNS) regulation of, 15*fig*; sympathetic
nervous system (SNS) regulation of, 15*fig*
salt-and-pepper bath, 134–36
Sarah's story, 29–31
*Science in the Art of osteopathy: Osteopathic
Principles and Practice* (Stone), 13
sea buckthorn, 147
self-awareness development, 62, 65
self-care techniques: positive emotion, 54,
102, 155–73, 195–202, 205; positive function, 54, 95–101, 138–52, 184–89*table*;
positive motion, 52, 54, 74, 76–83, 102,

self-care techniques: positive emotion (cont.) 153–54, 193–95; positive structure, 54, 85–95, 120–28, 182–84

self-healing trigger points: for anger, 126table, 129table, 244; for anxiety and depression, 125table, 129table, 244; benefits of using your, 121–22; for colds and coughs, 246; for hangovers, 247; for headaches, 129table, 248; how to apply, 122; illustration of the body's, 123; instructions for working with specific, 124table–29table; for lower back pain, 126table, 127table, 128table, 249; for low libido, 127table, 129table, 250; for menstrual pain, 251; for neck pain, 252; for thyroid problems, 254; for travel and jet lag, 255. See also myofacial trigger points; Positive Feedback remedies

self-talk: negative, 61; positive, 103–7

Seligman, Martin, 198

sexual assault victims, 165

shame psychological antidote, 60

shiitake mushrooms, 148

shingles, 4, 25

Short-Grain Brown Rice or Quinoa, 236

showering: alternating hot and cold rinses, 182–83; silent prayer while, 133. See also baths

side dish recipes: Black-Eyed Peas, 239; Chickpea Salad, 241–42; French Green Beans, 238; Garlic and Chili Broccolini (Long-Stem Broccoli), 237–38; Guacamole, 242; Peas and Artichoke Hearts, 239–40; Short-Grain Brown Rice or Quinoa, 236; Speltotto (Pearled-Spelt Risotto), 234–36; Spinach and Rice, 236–37; Steamed Asparagus with Lemon, 237; Sweet Potato Mash, 241; White Beans with Cinnamon, 240. See also vegetables

silent prayer, 133

skeletal health, 20

skin issues: as common reason for seeking medical help, 11; how diet can contribute to, 45; inflammatory foods associated with, 140. See also eczema

sleep: biological importance of, 72; consequences of chronic deprivation of, 72; daily naps, 136–38, 192; getting sufficient amount of quality, 72–73; tips for ensuring quality, 73–75

sleep problems: consequences of chronic, 72; inflammatory foods associated with, 140; Positive Feedback To-Go Plan for improving, 192; self-healing trigger points to help improve, 126table, 128, 129table

smoking, 19

smoothies: Liver Flush Smoothie, 144–45; Radiate Meal Plan recipes for, 218table–19table; suggested breakfast, 101

snacks: Positive Feedback To-Go Plan on, 192; Radiate Meal Plan, 216table–17table, 221table; Release (Days 1–3) Liver Flush, 143; Release (Days 1–7), 213table

Socrates, 56

sore throat remedies, 253–54

soup recipes: Pumpkin (or Sweet potato) Soup, 227; Village Soup, 227–28

soy beans, 149

soy products, 149

soy sauce, 149

Speltotto (Pearled-Spelt Risotto), 234–36

spice sensitivities, 152

Spinach and Rice, 236–37

spinal column "decoder ring," 13

spleen, 9

Stanton Peele Addiction Center, 158

Steamed Asparagus with Lemon, 237

Still, Andrew Taylor, 3, 51, 52, 54

stomach: parasympathetic nervous system (PNS) regulation of, 15fig; sympathetic nervous system (SNS) regulation of, 15fig

Stone, Caroline, 13, 26

stress: Adaptive Response growing stronger because of, 18; constantly tapping into Adaptive Response to handle daily, 56; how the Adaptive Response develops a greater resistance to, 54–55; how both Positive and Negative Feedback start in moment of, 52; impact on the HPA axis by chronic, 16–17; Maladaptive Response to, 18–19; Negative Feedback due to unmanaged, 20; when triggering stress becomes a default condition, 21–22. See also post-traumatic stress disorder

structure self-care techniques, description of, 54

Sucralose (Splenda), 151–52

sugared foods: candy, 149; cereals, 149

sulforaphane, 143

supplements, 215

Sweet Potato Mash, 241

sympathetic nervous system (SNS): being ruled by our, 60; description of, 14; heavily influenced by thoughts, 20; list of typical of daily SNS triggers, 17; regulation of functioning organs by, 15fig; wear and tear of emotional triggers impacting the, 16–19, 21. See also autonomic nervous system

Take a Nap! Change Your Life (Mednick and Ehrman), 137

tangerines, 148

Team in Training (Leukemia and Lymphoma Society), 194

teas: chamomile, 73, 222table; healing, 222table

tequila, 222table

Thieves Oil, 253
thyroid remedies, 254
Tibetan Rites: consider adding to evening routine, 74; deep breathing exercise to finish the, 83; history of the, 77; illustrations of the five rites of, 78–82; lymphatic fluids released during the, 52; Morning Glory ritual (Radiate phase), 182; Morning Glory ritual (Reflect phase), 76, 78–82; Morning Glory ritual (Release phase), 130; positive motion of the, 102; Radiate phase and expanding the, 194
Time Audit: description and purpose of the, 107–8; Kerry's story on her, 116–17; Release the Time-Wasters exercise, 117, 156–58; template for, 106*table*–7*table*
TMAO, 150
tomatoes, 149
tomato juice, 149
trauma: Body Timeline to recall painful, 94–95; EMDR therapy to release memory of, 162, 164–66; Negative Feedback due to unresolved childhood, 20; "post-traumatic growth" following, 53–54. *See also* pain
travel/jet lag: dietary suggestions for, 256–57; other remedies for, 255–56; self-healing trigger points for, 255
Tropical Smoothie, 218*table*
tummy massage, 182, 183–84
tumor necrosis factor, 73
Type 2 diabetes, 59, 214

University of California, San Diego, 137
University of Chicago study, 61
University of Pennsylvania, 198
University of Texas, 165
upper back pain: Adam's story on his, 33–35; common profile of, 31–35; physical and emotional causes of, 27*fig*; self-healing trigger points to help with, 129*table*
urinary tract infections, 184

Valerian root capsules (*Valeriana officinalis*), 75
vegetable-based brushes, 131
vegetables: Positive Feedback, 189*table*; Positive Feedback protein sources in, 188*table*; Release Meal Plan, 213*table*; white potatoes, 149. *See also* side dish recipes
Vicodin overdoses, 12
Village Soup, 227–28
vinegars, 149
visualization: create your release through meditation and, 163, 166–67; of forgiveness and release, 171–73; meditation for happiness, 205
vitamin B complex, 247

vitamin C, 77, 247, 257
vitamin D, 204
vitamin D deficiency, 20
Vlachonis, Vicky: analyzing the whole picture, 47–50; learning the power of food to hurt or heal during childhood, 41–43; turnaround from PCOS pain to health, 43–47
vodka, 149, 222*table*

Wake Forest University study, 109
walking exercise, 153–54, 192
Warrior Smoothie, 218*table*
water retention: inflammatory foods associated with, 140; self-healing trigger points in case of, 128*table*
Wellspring Institute for Neuroscience and Contemplative Wisdom, 60
wheat products, 149
whiplash, 32
whiskey, 149
White Beans with Cinnamon, 240
white potatoes, 149
white vegetables, 189*table*
worry: linkage between lungs and, 9; SNS triggered by overwork and, 120

yellow/orange fruits and vegetables, 189*table*
yin and yang, 129*table*
yoga, 154
yogurt (live), 187*table*

Zoe's story, 196–97

SCAN THIS CODE
WITH YOUR SMARTPHONE TO BE LINKED TO
THE BONUS MATERIALS FOR

THE BODY DOESN'T LIE

on the Elixir website,
where you can also find information about other
healthy living books and related materials.

YOU CAN ALSO TEXT

BODYPAIN to READIT (732348)

to be sent a link to the Elixir website.

 Facebook.com/elixirliving   Twitter.com/elixirliving   www.elixirliving.com